D1384336

Our Gift of Love

Personal Stories of Breast Cancer Courage

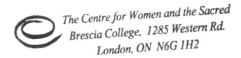

The Centre for Women and the Sacred
Brescia College, 1285 Western Rd.
London, ON N6G 1H2

GIBBS·SMITH
P
PUBLISHER

Salt Lake City

First edition
00 99 98 97 96   5 4 3 2 1

This is a Peregrine Smith Book, published by
Gibbs Smith, Publisher
P.O. Box 667
Layton, Utah 84041

Design by Kristin Bernhisel-Osborn

Photograph on front cover by Mike Rothwell. Courtesy of The Stock Solution, Salt Lake City, Utah.

Interior photographs courtesy of Brian Twede, Salt Lake City, Utah.

Printed and bound in the United States

Library of Congress Cataloging-in-Publication Data
Our gift of love : personal stories of breast cancer courage. — 1st ed.
        p. cm.
     "A Peregrine Smith book"—T.p. verso.
     Includes bibliographical references.
     ISBN 0-87905-791-2
     1. Breast—Cancer—Patients—Biography.
     RC280.B8086 1996
     362.1'9699449—dc20   96-33484
                                         CIP

About the cover: Cheryl Defa, a friend of the contributors, suggested in her self-penned obituary that her friends not mourn for her passing but instead plant a pink tulip as a remembrance. Our cover tulip, with its delicate petals and sturdy bulb, symbolizes the taproot of strength hidden beneath the surface in all of us.

Hollister & Company is a group of survivors who have had breast cancer. Led by Karen Johnson, Missy Cannell, Sherry Drabner, and Marie Knowles, the group represents thirty-one authors.

To Hugh Hollister Hogle, M.D.

You are the strength behind our words.
You gave us inspiration to write from our hearts.
We thank you and give you *Our Gift of Love.*

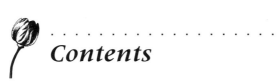

Contents

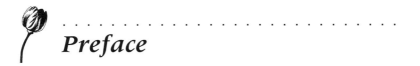

Preface

Why we wrote this book

Cancer is a scary word. No one wants to hear it.

Breast cancer is a scary disease. One in eight women will face it at some time.

And this is, in some ways, a scary book. It details the distress and disruption caused in perfectly normal lives when a group of cells launches itself on a course of rampant imperialism.

The authors—the women themselves, their husbands, children, parents, and health-care providers—recount the physical realities of surgery, chemotherapy, and radiation therapy. They speak of the emotional shock of finding the cancer, the spiritual struggle of facing mutilation and potential death. They describe the impact of cancer on family and friends, as well as the changes that diagnosis and treatment inevitably bring.

But this book is also a reassuring book, a hopeful book. The authors express not only the anguish and anger of having breast cancer enter their lives but also the process of coming to terms with the disease, the human solidarity that arises when a loved one is in danger, the strength that comes from facing the upheaval and the fear. It is a how-to book, a manual for survival, a plan for using the disease as a springboard to a more consciously lived life.

Because the authors were free to focus on what was most important to them, there are several themes that appear in many of the stories: discovery of the disease, surgery and recovery, the effects of chemotherapy and radiation therapy, personal fear and grief, the search for information, family reactions, family history of cancer, support groups, spiritual and emotional help from religion and from books, insurance problems, the need for more research and political action, handling the fear of recurrence, and living with actual recurrence or metastasis of the disease. These common aspects serve to highlight the very individual ways in which each person faces the threat and the challenge.

Although this book could have been organized in many ways, we chose to emphasize the fact that breast cancer doesn't only happen to the woman but also to her spouse, her family, her friends, her health-care providers, and other women with breast cancer. And in turn, a woman can look to some or all of those people for support.

We wrote this book partly for ourselves. It was a way to sort out and come to terms with the experience of having cancer, a way to tell the world, "This is what happened to me; this is where I am now." It was also a way to tell the people we love how important their support and participation was and is in our lives, to thank them for being there. But most of all, this book is a way to help others in the same circumstances, to show them what to expect physically and emotionally, and to give them courage and hope as well as practical information.

It is our gift of love.

Caira (Missy) Cannell and Elizabeth Hansen
Sherry Drabner
Bridget Feighan
Joy Feist
Cindy Friend and Randall Friend
Peggy Hatch
Hugh H. Hogle
Roxann Glassey and John Glassey
Roberta James
Karen J. Johnson and Tricia Paxton Warnock
Marie Carnesecca Knowles

Loraine Lovell
K. Mack and Tim Rule
Dian Mahin
Ann Martin
Vicki Mickelsen and David Mickelsen
Betty R. Pittman
Joy Rogers
Beverley Seale
Barbara Thayne Green and Alisyn Thayne
Susan Cambigue-Tracey and Paul Tracey
Doreen Weyland
Val C. Wilcox
Stephanie Zimmer

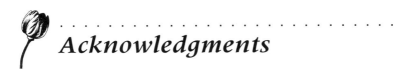

Acknowledgments

Special thanks to Dr. Hugh H. Hogle for having the vision; Mikale DesJardins for assisting with typing and her enthusiasm and faith in this book; Professor Stephen R. Baar for his suggestions and encouragement; Professor Patricia Aikins Coleman for her grammar corrections and excitement for this project; all the doctors, nurses, friends, and family who have encouraged us to follow our dream to complete this book to share with the world; Richard Paul Evans for his love and belief that this book was an important venture and worthy of inclusion on his goal list; Leslie Smith, R.N., for gathering medical sketches; Vicki Mickelson for her endless hours of editing; Joy Feist for her support for the financial beginnings of this book; Doreen Weyland for her long hours of editing assistance; the Breast Cancer Coalition for sponsoring the 1993 March to Washington, D.C., where the beginnings of Hollister and Company were formed; Shirley Rossa, M.S.W., for inspiring women to write their own obituaries; Cheryl Defa for writing her obituary asking people to plant a pink tulip to remember women touched by breast cancer; Fred Oswald for creatively suggesting the purchase of a bench surrounded by pink tulips at the Red Butte Arboretum; Brian Twede for his photography; Chris Vanocur, who believed in the book and created a television program based on its premise for Mother's Day 1995 (nominated for an Emmy); Marie Carnesecca Knowles, Sherry Drabner, and Missy Cannell for encouraging, financially supporting, and seeing this work to completion; and Karen Johnson for never letting the dream die. Very special thanks to all those at Gibbs Smith, Publisher—especially Theresa Desmond—who had patience and appreciation for this important work.

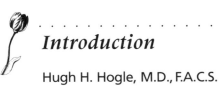

Introduction

Hugh H. Hogle, M.D., F.A.C.S.

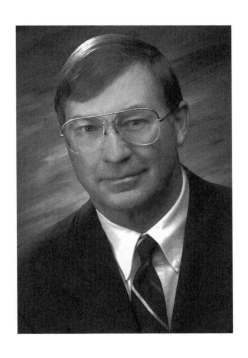

Hugh Hogle graduated from the University of Utah Medical School and subsequently interned at UCLA Harbor General Hospital. He then returned to Utah to complete a general surgery residency. For fifteen years, he practiced general surgery in Salt Lake City at Holy Cross Hospital and during that time was actively involved in the care of many women with breast diseases. His interest in breast pathology and breast diseases led him to develop and establish the first Breast Care Center in the intermountain west at Holy Cross Hospital.

After 1987, he limited his practice to diseases and surgery of the breast. He was the director of Breast Care Services *at St. Mark's Hospital in Salt Lake City. He has been actively involved in breast-cancer research and has served on numerous local and national breast-care-related boards. He has been the recipient of the American Cancer Society's Sword of Hope Award. Dr. Hogle and his wife, Carol, have six children.*

On January 15, 1995, while fishing in Brazil, Dr. Hogle suffered a stroke. He is no longer practicing medicine. Today he works in the four retail fishing stores owned by the family. He finds pleasure in hunting, fishing, photography, and spending time with his family.

This is a book about breast cancer. It has been written by those who have experienced the disease and by their loved ones.

Some of its authors are dying of the disease. Others may still harbor the lethal cells and not yet know their fate. Two-thirds are probably "cured."

I have had the privilege to care for many of the authors, but some have had their care rendered by other physicians.

There are other books written by women who have had breast cancer. Most are by a single author; several are written by multiple authors. This book is a tapestry woven by many individual experiences. It is their story. It will make you laugh, and it will make you cry. It will inspire you and anger you. But most of all, it will teach you.

This book was written for women with newly diagnosed breast cancer, but its lessons are universal. No one who reads this book will be untouched.

I was asked to write about the physician's perspective on breast cancer and the women who face the challenge of this disease. I considered a didactic approach dealing with the biology of the disease and all of the risks and benefits of the various modern treatment options and modalities. This information is readily available from multiple excellent sources (such as *Dr. Susan Love's Breast Book*), and, therefore, I elected another approach that is substantially more personal, and, for me, significantly more difficult.

In 1972, I was chief surgical resident at the University of Utah Medical Center. One afternoon while we were making rounds, I was paged overhead. It was my father. The minute I heard his voice, I knew there was a problem because he would never call me at the hospital unless it was a matter of urgency.

"Your mother has a breast lump." His voice was tense.

"Let me talk to her," I answered. My mother came on the phone and explained that she had found a lump in her right breast while she was taking a shower. As my mother has always done, she trivialized the significance of her find. She has always underplayed personal health issues. Perhaps it is a form of denial, but I sense that it operates more as a protection for her loved ones than a real denial process.

We both said reassuring things to one another, and I told her I would make arrangements for her to see one of our faculty staff surgeons the next day. I found Dr. Maxwell, and he agreed to see her the following afternoon.

My mother was fifty-four years old. She was just beginning to enter menopause and looked at least ten years younger than her chronological age. She grew up a few decades before the diet and exercise era, but she had maintained a slender, healthy physique and never weighed an ounce more than 110 pounds. We had no breast-cancer history in our family, her first son was born when she was twenty-one, and there were no other breast-cancer risk factors.

We finished rounds, and I went home since I was off duty that evening. Driving home, I kept remembering a statement I had heard my mother make on numerous occasions: "If I ever get breast cancer, I will not let them remove my breast." At our house, we did not talk much about personal "things," and so her statement about her breasts had had a somewhat startling and profound impact upon me. What would she do if the lump turned out to be a cancer? The only acceptable option in 1972 was mastectomy. But hey! Only one lump in ten turns out to be breast cancer, and that happens to other people's families.

The next day, she saw Dr. Maxwell, and a biopsy under local anesthesia was scheduled for the following day. I stopped by to see her the evening before surgery, and again we said reassuring things; but I palpated the lump through her clothing, and I left her home that evening anything but reassured. Her lump was firm, not movable.

The biopsy had been scheduled for 11:00 A.M., but it was past 1:00 P.M. when they wheeled her into the operating room. As a surgeon nearing the end of his training, I had been involved in hundreds of operations, but her operating room seemed as alien and strange as it had the first time I had been in the surgical suite as a medical student. I had performed many breast biopsies in this same O.R., but that day I would be only an observer. I was uncertain whether I wanted to be there at all.

We made structured, uneasy small talk as Dr. Maxwell removed the formless piece of whitish-yellow breast tissue, which contained the jelly-bean-sized mass in its center. After the lump was removed, one of the surgical lights was pointed to the back table, and with a separate surgical blade the specimen was divided in half. The eyes above our masked faces said that her worst nightmare was coming true. The tan, spiculated, 1½-centimeter lesion was most certainly a cancer.

We strained to make small talk as her biopsy site was closed, and I am certain she felt and knew what we had found long before the pathologist called her report in to the room. She had received no sedation and could hear her surgeon talking to the pathologist. Dr. Maxwell listened intently for a few moments.

Then he said, "You're sure, absolutely sure?" Dr. Maxwell handed me the phone, and the pathologist repeated to me what my mother already knew.

"Bonnie, it's breast cancer." A single tear welled up in the corner of her eye and ran down toward her ear.

"Remember our conversation yesterday about the mastectomy?" Dr. Maxwell said softly.

She nodded affirmatively. She was still covered with surgical drapes but turned her head to look at me. I took her face in my hands and put my cheek close to hers.

"I said I would never do this."

"I know, Mom," I whispered.

For a few moments, we remained silent. Then I said, "Mom, you've got to do it. We don't have any other choices."

She nodded but said nothing. Again, a few moments passed in silence.

"Mom, let's get it over with."

She was silent for a moment more, then with a surprising air of resolve, she said, "Okay. Take it off. Let's get it over with."

I whispered that I loved her and stayed while the anesthesiologist reduced her to the dreamless sleep of general anesthesia, and then I left the room.

The corridor outside the operating room was littered with gurneys, carts, anesthesia machines, and the other assorted paraphernalia of surgery, but no one was in the hall. I slipped into the darkened anesthesia supply room and buried my face in a pillow and sobbed. I had just convinced my mother to do the one thing she had said she would never do. The shock of her cancer was terrible enough, but I also felt as if I had completely deserted her when she needed me most.

When I finally regained a modicum of composure, I went to find my father. He was in the waiting room, and if the long delay had not already confirmed his fears, my expression left no doubt. We embraced briefly and, while choking back tears, I told him what was underway. He assured me that she was doing the right thing. It helped, but not much.

Her recovery was exactly what I would have expected of her.

She made everything return to normal overnight, and, to this day, I do not know how she felt about doing the only thing she said she would "never do." It has been nineteen years, and she is alive and well and rarely mentions breast cancer. Most of the family have almost forgotten she ever had the disease. I know that she thinks about it every single day.

Following the completion of my surgical training, I remained at the University Hospital, thinking that a career in the academic setting would be suited to my interests. The technical part of surgery and patient care have always been my medical priorities, but teaching and research have also interested me. After my first year on the surgical faculty, however, I found I was doing more administrative tasks and not enough patient care or surgery to satisfy my professional goals. I decided to leave the University and enter solo private practice. I joined the surgical staff of Holy Cross Hospital in Salt Lake City, Utah. Holy Cross is a middle-sized nonprofit hospital, owned and operated by the Sisters of the Holy Cross. There were nine other general surgeons on the hospital's active staff, and I knew and had worked with all of them during my residency training. All of them treated me well, and most shared their emergency-room coverage with me. In a matter of a few months, I was as busy as any young surgeon could have hoped to be.

During the first four or five years of my practice, I saw my share of patients with breast problems and breast cancer. My mother's experience undoubtedly affected my approach and empathy for women with breast diseases.

As my experience with breast cancer increased, it became evident that early detection was critical to a favorable outcome with this disease. More and more data from major studies also supported this conclusion. Based on this information, I devised an organizational scheme to establish a dedicated breast-care center at our hospital. The major focus of the center would be the promotion of early detection of breast cancer through increased use of mammography, clinical breast examination, and teaching breast self-examination. These services would be actively encouraged through public education and marketing. In the original proposal, which I presented in 1976 to the administration of the hospital, the center would also accept self-referred patients and would provide not only screening and education but also after-care services such as patient and family counseling, support groups, and psychological and physical rehabilitation.

The hospital administration liked the idea, and the Medical Staff Executive Committee approved the proposal; but for reasons that are unimportant now, the Breast Care Center's gestation period was almost eight years from conception to its birth in 1984. Had it not been for the dynamic support of Sisters Suzanne Brennan and Margo Cain, Holy Cross's Breast Care Center might still be no more than a proposal at the bottom of a pile of papers gathering dust on some vice president's desk.

Since the center's inception, the number of women utilizing its services and the variety of services have grown with each passing year. Breast diagnostic studies have gone from about 2,000 in 1983 to approximately 22,000 in 1991. Much of this growth can be attributed to the compassionate expertise of the breast care provided by our nursing and technical staff. Some of the growth, however, is related to increasing national awareness and emphasis upon the importance of breast-cancer screening by agencies such as the American College of Surgeons and the American College of Radiologists.

Because of my association with the Breast Care Center and my interest in breast cancer, my surgical practice underwent a natural evolution. Over time, I did more breast-related care and fewer other general surgical procedures. Finally, I decided to limit my practice to diseases and surgery of the breast. This concentration of surgical practice, study, research, and interest has provided a unique opportunity to experience a level of involvement in breast care that is not usually available in most general surgical practices. The intensity of my breast-related practice has resulted in my being involved with a large number of women whose cancers have taught me valuable lessons.

The human impact and the complexities of breast cancer are both intriguing and constantly challenging. The uncertainties of the disease and the burdens of its treatment impose dramatic hardships upon the afflicted. Those who would treat this disease must be prepared for failure. The realization that one out of four women who present for breast-cancer care is going to die is a stressful and sobering thought. For the treating surgeon, the task of informing someone that her biopsy has shown a breast cancer never, never becomes painless. Watching those you have come to know and to care for endure the ordeal of terminal breast cancer is frustrating, dispiriting, and painful.

Although the rendering of care to breast-cancer patients has its share of lows, the privilege of being associated with the courageous women who valiantly battle this silent enemy has been a constant source of inspiration.

The chapters that follow are their stories. Every year over 185,000 American women will write new chapters. It is the hope of all of us who work in the struggle against this disease that monthly breast self-examination, annual professional breast examination, and mammography can help ensure that these chapters will have a happy ending.

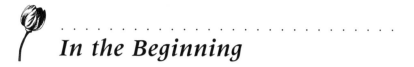

In the Beginning

The stories in this chapter represent two of the ways women have come to terms with the experience of breast cancer.

The first is a letter that actually initiated the idea for this book. It is a look at the experience after the event by a woman who has thought carefully and deeply about its effects on her life.

The second is a collection of poetry written as the author went through the stages of diagnosis, surgery, and treatment. Although many of the authors have included poems in their stories, in this case the poetry *is* the story.

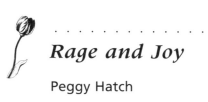

Rage and Joy

Peggy Hatch

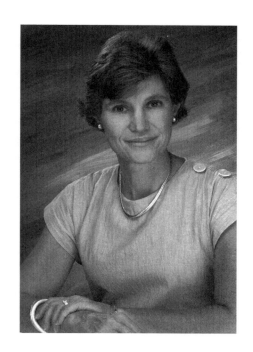

Peggy Hatch was born in Vienna, Austria, and immigrated to the United States at age three. She met her husband of twenty-five years, Jeff, at Stanford University. Subsequently, Peggy received her Ph.D. in counseling psychology. Life is satisfying with her three adored children and fulfilling profession. "Playtime" includes traveling, reading, friends, volunteer work, gardening, and almost any imaginable outdoor activity.

Medical Bio

During the summer of 1988, Peggy noticed a small lump in the upper inner quadrant of her left breast. As she followed it for several months, it seemed to decrease in size. In September, an examination revealed a 1.2-centimeter firm lump at the 10 o'clock position, just beyond the edge of her areola. A needle aspiration of the lump revealed atypical cells, but malignancy was not identified. Because the lump was solid, she was scheduled for a breast biopsy. The subsequent pathology revealed the presence of a 1.1-centimeter invasive breast cancer.

Following extensive consultation, Peggy elected to be treated with conservation therapy, and in November 1988 she underwent reexcision of her biopsy site, and the lymph glands were removed from her left armpit. None of them contained any metastatic tumor. She went through six weeks of radiation therapy to her left breast with a total dose of 5,040 rads (radiation absorbed dose). Following her recuperation from the surgery and radiation, she began adjuvant chemotherapy. She did not complete the anticipated course of chemotherapy and at this time is healthy with no evidence of recurrent disease.

February 10, 1990

Dear Hugh,

Thank you for inviting me to your breast-cancer conference. It afforded me the rare luxury of time to reflect on . . . what? . . . life, really. I'm a bit removed from the "heat of the battle" with cancer at this time so can be somewhat dispassionate.

I have almost never regretted the experience of having had breast cancer. In fact, with some embarrassment, I confided to my closest friends my frequent thought that having had cancer was one of the best experiences of my life. It has certainly been one of the most significant, along with leaving home, falling in love with my husband, letting go of and burying my father, and giving birth to my children and watching them grow.

Before I had cancer, I suffered from intermittent bouts with depression. My husband and I were engaged in debilitating squabbles. I was too little involved in my own life and too much involved in the lives of my friends. Only my work and my children left me with a sense of wholeness and satisfaction. But since my diagnosis, I have felt a joy and an intensity about living that is difficult to comprehend. Two years later, I miraculously still feel wonderful with no further depressive symptoms.

I am no Pollyanna. Often I am sad and cry when I look at my poor, maimed breasts. It is not vanity that makes me weep but sadness at life's inexorable movement towards death, symbolized by the scars across my chest. It's not really any different than realizing that I have become invisible to most men, no longer being young and "cute," or that it takes a Herculean effort to keep up with my eleven-year-old on the basketball court. It's not different in substance but in its dramatic intensity. We can ignore many little signs in our everyday world that life will end, whether with a bang or a whimper, but breast cancer is impossible to ignore.

We run around to doctors who cut us, irradiate us, strip us naked, poke us with needles, and make us sick. They force us to face our mortality, even when they are most kind and supportive. I am thankful for them, even when I rage at their insensitivity, their narrow focus on their specialty (which paradoxically is exactly what we hire them for), and their struggles about facing our mutual knowledge of life's tenuousness. (For the most part, I chose my doctors well. They had the courage to deal with me as a human being, not merely as a breast cancer.)

I hate the word *grateful,* yet I'm grateful for the opportunity that breast cancer gave me to face death, to know death, to feel death in me; I believe it is only by being intimate with death that we can choose life and love. Mythology and religion express this part of ourselves. The phoenix rises from the ashes. Christ, crucified, rises from the dead to save mankind, to give life to mankind. For me, breast cancer has been a similar and very humbling experience, a rebirth, a transformation. I more deeply appreciate my loved ones. The small things in life that used to irritate me have lost much of their significance, even though I'm still the same kind of fussy, perfectionist person that drives others nuts. More importantly, I cherish every moment of life. I love my "babies" and am more patient with the real person who is my husband. I appreciate each sunny day, each rainy day, the heat, the cold, even the feel of my pillow on my face as I go to bed at night. What a gift breast cancer has been!

During the conference you asked me what allowed me to get over my anger about my situation. I responded rather facilely that I got over my anger by taking control of my life. Although my response was accurate, it didn't sound quite right when I said it; it was incomplete.

Coming to terms with breast cancer meant coming to terms not only with death but with myself: who I am in an essential way, what matters to me, what values I hold. In a sense, I came to know myself more wholly—I could not avoid this in the usual way by hiding behind conventionality, social roles, and habit. None of those external standards matter anymore in the same way.

I learned that life, per se, matters little to me, that I care about the quality of life, not the quantity. I relearned how important it is for me to feel in control of the parts of my life that I *do* have a say about. Paradoxically, I simultaneously realized that some mythical notion of "I'm in charge" isn't necessary. I also learned that I don't feel that having cancer was being singled out for punishment by the gods; I believe that the universe is a rather arbitrary place.

It is currently very fashionable to believe that we can control disease and life itself by our attitudes, by what we eat, think, and do. Although there may be some truth to these ideas, I think they can be enormously destructive. I do not think it is "good for my health" to think that I caused my cancer because I was depressed or because of any other attitude of mine. A funny article by Russell Baker in the *New York Times Magazine* addressed this. Baker said he was glad that he wouldn't be able to attend his own funeral because he was certain that all his friends would blame him for his own death, saying that he ate the wrong food, didn't exercise enough, was too stressed, kept the wrong company, etc. I have yet to meet the human being who wasn't going to die of something, and I believe many of these attitudes spring from our reluctance to deal with our mortality.

I came once again to terms with something I had learned years ago in therapy—that I'm responsible for myself even when I can't control my circumstances. I believe Marcus Aurelius's old philosophical notion that it is not events themselves that disturb men, but the view that they hold of them. I also relearned another of life's lessons—that we are never done until we're dead. As time goes on, I respond differently to my diagnosis. Even today, its meaning to me continues to change.

I wasn't at all worried about having cancer in the first place. You were very reassuring. You said, "Probably just a cyst." (It wasn't. The lump didn't aspirate.) "Negative mammogram." (It was negative, both two years before cancer and at the time I discovered the lump staring at me in the mirror.) "Ninety-five-percent chance it's just a fibroma; doesn't feel like breast cancer." (It was a rather hard, well-defined lump.) "Cytology negative, though you do seem to have some proliferation of cells." (No cancer cells in the sample, but more cells than normal; a common phenomenon, but often cancerous or precancerous.) "Still, we need to take it out and look at it." (Cancer, after all.)

I've always been interested in almost anything around me, including the biopsy—I wasn't the slightest bit worried. In fact, I wanted to have a local and watch the whole process and was very disappointed when my view was obscured by a drape put in front of my face to prevent my contaminating the "field" by breathing on my breast. I was a little like the folks who took picnic baskets up on the hillsides to watch the first battles of the Civil War.

I had no inkling of my own anxiety until my husband showed up, slightly late and breathless, in the recovery area. Today I still feel ashamed and a bit superstitious that I yelled at him, "You don't care! I hope it's breast cancer, and I hope it's spread to my lungs!" (Someone once told me that the worst curse one could inflict upon another was to make his or her wish come true.) I'd not made any big deal about his being there earlier, acting as low-key and cheerfully curious with him as with myself.

I didn't experience any fear when you told me I had breast cancer. I just blandly said, "Well, now what? Do we chop it off or what?" Fortunately, you wouldn't let me get away with such a cold-blooded approach. You forced me to think about and deal with the implications of any treatment I chose.

Once in gear, I did my obsessive-compulsive thing and read everything I could get my hands on. I consulted with my physician friends and their physician friends across the country, collecting opposing opinions, research, and philosophies of treatment. My way of understanding these issues, which hinged on a technical education far beyond any training I would ever have, was to pit one doctor's views against the next. Whichever appeared to make the most sense, both medically and personally, was what I implemented at that moment for my own treatment.

If I were to give you a bottom line of what I learned from all my inquiries, it would be this: "We really know very little about breast cancer. We know very little about effective treatment. We change our minds every few months about the best treatment for any specific manifestation of the disease. We can make some reasonable guesses about who will get well and who won't, but they're only guesses. Our treatments are probably better most of the time than no treatment, taking into account economic, social, psychological, and medical factors. Finally, the earlier you are diagnosed and cared for medically and personally, the better your odds of living, taking into account heredity and tumor characteristics."

When I went to consult with my oncologist for the first time, I was armed with two pages of questions on my yellow legal pad. I listened to his spiel with half an ear—it was already old information and much too general. When I finished with him an hour later, he teased me about putting him through his board exams again. We laughed together, but he wouldn't let me leave until I'd told him whether he had passed or failed. He passed, poor man. He has a challenging job, and I suspect that though I was a cheerful patient, I was provocative and difficult throughout treatment. I "tested" him more than once.

I think because I informed myself and took control of my treatment, I felt less helpless about coping with an arbitrary, catastrophic event in my life. I chose the treatment that made the best sense to me at the time. I was a candidate for, and opted for, lumpectomy and radiation treatment with six months of chemotherapy. I'm still a bit anxious about the radiation treatment's possible long-term cancer-inducing potential but was not yet ready to lose my breast if I didn't have to. I'm not certain that I would choose chemotherapy again. The National Cancer Institute had just released the recommendation, based on incomplete data, that non-negative, stage-1 breast cancers be treated with chemotherapy. Most doctors I consulted with felt bound by the recommendation but were angry with the political nature of the report. Many felt it was a funding ploy. Patients were the ball that was being batted around the political court. Nonetheless, I know I made as careful a choice about treatment as I could have, and have no regrets about my choice to this day.

I enjoyed my radiation treatments. I suffered no physical ill effects and appreciated the few moments of enforced "quiet time" during radiation when I could relax and meditate. It was also enjoyable to meet the father of a close college friend in the radiation waiting room—we cheered each other on. I planned my chemotherapy so that I could keep my regular work hours but so that I would still be in relatively good shape for the weekends. I stayed away from sick people, let myself rest, and made myself exercise daily, even when my normal run was reduced to a tired walk. I vomited only once, though I became quite irritable towards the end of my treatment. Regarding hair loss: I lost mostly pubic hair and remained defiantly determined to wear a purple wig if necessary.

I had decided to take charge of my experience with cancer and to live with it as gracefully as possible. For the most part, my approach worked well. My nature is to be in control. As with all of our natures, the very things that work for us also work against us. I didn't allow myself or others to nurture me, to feel any fear or insecurity or even anger until at least six months to a year after my diagnosis. Who wants to cry with you a year after the fact, when even the last signs of treatment have faded?

Independent of my "control" of the situation, my friends and family were there for me. They fed the kids and me, inquired about my well-being, and just generally made life easier. Often they felt helpless in the face of my persistent competence and the denial of fears, anxieties, or worries. I couldn't share their anxiety because I wasn't aware of my own anxiety at the time.

For me the most upsetting aspect of the cancer and the treatment was that partway through chemotherapy, the treatments threw me into premature menopause. Why did that affect me so? After all, many women are delighted to be done with all that. I was approaching menopause anyway, and my family was complete. It affected me for many reasons, it turns out, but mainly because I was unprepared. My intense study and consultation had been about breast cancer, not menopause. I read that chemotherapy caused "menstrual difficulties," but I didn't pursue the meaning of that in great detail. Menopause might occur 50 percent of the time, according to my doctor. Being healthy and relatively insensitive to drugs, I didn't expect that to be a problem for me—you know, the old self-centered notion that bad things only happen to other people, and only if they deserve it.

What I didn't know was that my likelihood of going into menopause was really 90 to 100 percent, given my age of forty-two. My doctors were concerned about curing cancer, not about something as trivial as menopause for a middle-aged woman with three children. I felt a bit ashamed when I initially challenged my doctor about what the books had meant by "menstrual difficulties" and he replied, "Isn't your family complete? Did you want more children?" Only later was I able to realize the full ramifications of menopause: the associated, demonstrable aging process involved, and the inadequate, non-estrogen means of coping with menopausal symptoms available to me. I wanted to go back to him with my rage and say something like, "Look, Doc, you don't want any more kids, do you? Why don't we just whack *your* thing off and give you one of those neato inflatable jobs—it does the same thing."

I began suffering the effects of menopause two-thirds of the way through my chemotherapy. I became depressed, though I didn't feel emotionally depressed. My memory became very disturbed. I found myself unable to think clearly and suffered a loss of energy. My skin and breasts sagged and aged precipitously. I lost my libido, and my vagina atrophied. Continuous hot flashes through the night left me sleepless and exhausted. I raged at everyone for this additional insult. I could be a brave soldier about the breast cancer, the surgeries, and the specifics I had expected of chemo. But I refused to take on menopause. I threw a six-month-long temper tantrum that included skipping the last two weeks of chemotherapy.

Part of my rage, I realized, was at the loss of innocence about life. Yes, cancer dramatically demonstrated that life could end, but menopause felt even worse because it so clearly depicted our inevitable and gradual physical deterioration. It also meant that dealing with cancer and the treatment for cancer couldn't ever "be over," even when the chemotherapy was done.

I did more research in my characteristic coping style, this time regarding menopause, estrogen-replacement therapy, and cancer. Information about menopause is easily obtained. Almost no information is available regarding actual studies comparing premenopausal women and breast cancer survival rates to postmenopausal cancer survival rates controlling for heredity, tumor characteristics, etc. Oophorectomies are no longer performed because they did not increase survival rates. It is known that estrogen "feeds" cancer cells, so medical advice and information is restricted to: "Estrogen replacement therapy (ERT) is not advised for women who have had breast cancer." I decided to take estrogen replacement therapy anyway, because I was willing to take a calculated risk that 1) all my cancer cells had been destroyed or 2) my immune system could handle any that remained. Few doctors would be willing to cooperate with my choice. With ERT my menopausal symptoms have disappeared and I am temporarily protected from the symptoms which would force further loss of innocence about aging. It is a protection I need for now, though I don't think I'm a fool about it.

I am still dealing with my fears about cancer in fits and starts. I've lost trust in my body. It betrayed me. There's no way to reassure me about my body anymore. I can't be comforted in the innocent belief that if I just behave, everything will be just fine. I am insecure and anxious about little aches, pains, and minor physical problems. Any slight tiredness that isn't accounted for, any soreness that shouldn't be there, and my anxiety escalates, along with shame. Am I just hypochondriacal? How can I tell? How will I ever be able to tell? The cancer. I ate enough vegetables to bloat Peter Rabbit. I don't drink much, don't smoke, don't eat many smoked meats, had my babies early, nursed them, and even picked relatives who didn't have breast cancer. It came anyway. Will it come again?

This spring I had a cervical polyp removed—no biggie. But I was terrified and trusted no one when they attempted to reassure me that the polyp was highly unlikely to be cancerous. It was one more thing. Doctors, hospitals, anesthesia, smells, and *uncertainty.*

I'm counterphobic in an attempt to reassure myself. Last summer we climbed the Grand Teton; this summer we're going river running. We just got back from mountain biking the Moab slickrock trail. My poor son finally asked why we couldn't have "normal" vacations like other people.

I'm sure there's more to come. Each day teaches me something new. The confrontation with death that cancer offers stimulates my zest for every particle of life. I cherish my fear, rage, and anger as much as my joy—it's all part of life and therefore fine with me. I'm happy to be involved in the process for as long as I'm able. In a sense, if we finally are able to accept anger, death, fear—those "shadow" parts of life that we're so reluctant to accept—and their negative attributes with grace, they simply become part of the whole of life and, as such, lose their sting.

It is my life. I may have had breast cancer, but how I respond to it, what I do with my life, is my choice. I choose for myself what I perceive to be a responsible, informed, quality life that I take charge of within the confines of nature and my fallible self, friends, doctors, and loves. Sometimes that is lonely, but it is my way. I have come to terms with who I am, the implications of the choices I make, what life means to me, and what I value. It is exciting to be able to make such life-and-death decisions. Thank you, Hugh, for being willing to participate with me throughout such an exciting process.

With affection,

Peggy Hatch

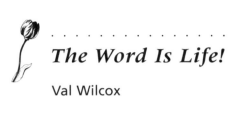

The Word Is Life!

Val Wilcox

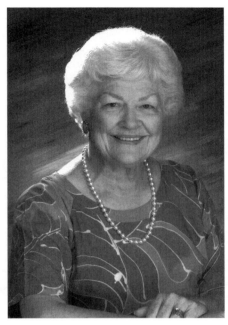

Val Camenish Wilcox and her husband are parents of four sons and grandparents of seventeen. They have traveled extensively and once lived for several years in Ethiopia, Africa. Val taught second grade for twenty years and is active in church and civic activities. Over the past twenty-five years Val has received many honors for her frequently published poems and lyrics. Her favorite things include cultivating people, enjoying Mexican food, sewing, and reading to her adored grandchildren.

Medical Bio

In the summer of 1987, while she was undergoing an evaluation for diabetes, Val had a screening mammogram that revealed a suspicious area in her left breast. A subsequent biopsy confirmed the diagnosis of infiltrating ductal carcinoma. She was sixty-two years old.

After considering the treatment options, she elected to have breast conservation and subsequently underwent the resection of the upper outer portion of her left breast and the surgical removal of her axillary lymph nodes. She then went through six weeks of radiation therapy to the left breast and a radiation boost to the area from which the tumor had been removed.

At this time, she has made a full recovery and is without evidence of breast cancer.

The Word Is Life!
Like a gladiator waiting
for his sign
from capricious power,
I cower in uncertainty.

Radiology finally sends
postoperative word
that I am cancer-free.
Thumbs up for me!

And Now I Vow
Here members of the family gather
to bless and comfort—
to help me overcome the sobbing fear
that no more years remain for me.

In answer to all prayers, a calm descends,
a peace of soul that cannot be described,
as I place self into the care of those
whose hands will do the cutting that can save.

Soon after drugged awakening comes the word
that pushes and expands life's boundaries.
And now I vow that ordinary days,
delivered every morning just on time,
will be received with purest gratitude
and constant joy!

Night Thoughts Before Surgery
Mastectomy—it rolls melodiously
as if it were a skateboard name
and not a cancer surgery.
I hate its raw intrusion in my life!

If I could
I would run from it
on lightning shoes.

I would thump away
in seven-league boots.

I would creep from it
on slippered feet
soundlessly
down hospital halls.

Perhaps I shall soon wear thongs
and walk in moist beach sand again.

Shapelessness of Shock
Like a pathetic pup
whimpering and licking wounds
of a just-lost fight,
she lay in a hospital bed
push-buttoned down.
Lying flat like that
she could see her uneven
body configuration—
right breast convex, as always,
but to the left
this new, unnatural cavity
taped with packings and tubes.

Though everyone exclaimed
over her good fortune
at finding the cancer so soon,
her head still whirled
at the speedy pace
of surgeon's, radiologist's
and loved ones' faces
floating through misty, buffered
places of drug-induced reality.
Too-serious changes came
too fast—and were the last
of how things used to be.

The Chosen One
To me, it is a mystery
Why God's chosen people
Have a history of abuse.

Now I am the chosen one—
One in ten, statistics say.*

Can I handle such an honor?
Do I even want to be
So select a person
This disease would come to me?

With all frantic "if's" and "maybe's"
My panic would be evident
Except for the crystalline calm of knowing
The promised land where I am going.

Putting Affairs in Order
Despite dismal prognosis
That narrows my future
To an imminent demise,
I will go to work as always
To do and try, to get and give,
Not living now to die,
But dying now to live!

Love Letter to Life
The test results are in
And like some secret sin,
This cancer deep within me now devours.
My time is measured here in days and hours,
As time has always been.

Some folks may curse their birth
If placed upon this earth

....
*The current (1996) statistic is that one in eight women will have breast cancer.

In hopelessness, in need and poverty,
Yet, never having known such misery,
I love this goodly earth.

So much I must achieve
That though I do believe
In afterlife where promises await,
YOU, world and lively life, in spite of fate—
YOU, I am loathe to leave.

I Do Have Need
(I Cor. 12:21)
"The eye cannot say unto the hand,
I have no need of thee."
I have high concern
about strange turns of fate
that find me waiting for surgery.
Every part has served the whole,
but who can tell what lab report
may now dictate for my body
and perhaps my soul?

X-ray Picture
On brightened screen,
Like a firework starburst
Captured on stop-action film,
Is a full-face shot
Of cell exploding
Out of normalcy
Into one gross cluster
Putting out tenacious feelers—
Malignancy!

Ugliness disguised
In flower beauty
Is still intent
Upon destructive duty.

Oncology Treatment Center
At first it seemed sufficient just to sit
and fill in those blank spaces on the forms,
but soon I looked around the room to see
this board game set up ready to be played
by equally blank faces waiting, too.

I find I am a player in this group
of folks who gather without fail each day
to play games no one wants, but none dare miss.
We never greet each other by our names—
we have no common interests or skills,
yet every day we meet at three-fifteen
to make our moves by thumbing magazines,
rechecking watches and avoiding eyes.

As our turns come we rise and disappear
through double doors to a labyrinth of halls
where science-fiction "zap" machines await
and measured radiation is applied.
This game of chance might be entitled "Life,"
"The Price is High" or "Jeopardy" or "Risk."
We play game pieces, mostly chemo tubes
and zaps, without the calculated odds.

To break the silent strain and even laugh,
my impulse is to roar right through these doors.
But no, I follow protocol and go
to meekly seek attention for my need,
yet never mentioning that dreadful word—
the reason we all came to play this game.

Radiation Therapy

As in some wide-screen space fantasy
I am here surrounded by
a phalanx of shiny machines,
nearly bare of clothing
and totally bereft of modesty
while white lab-coated others
use their tools to measure,
prod and mark.

Now, alone where silence rules
except for periodic whirrs,
I lie rigidly, exactly placed
for invisible rays
to work their healing magic
on what might have been
a tragic condition.

How I praise God
and bless all learned doctors
and technicians.
Also, within my mind and heart,
I honor Pierre and Marie Curie
whose dedicated searching
brought to be
the radiation therapy
now used in saving me.

One Size Fits All

Post-operative arm can't be raised yet,
And bruises look yellow and brown.
It took two of us fifty minutes
To clothe me and drive into town.
I dress up to go to the doctor,
Then undress to put on this gown.

Phantom Foe
Pervasive fear hovers
Over nebulous battlefield
Here in my body.
But will I ever even see
My phantom foe?

My impulse is to make impassioned charge
Impaling this antagonist
With poison dart through heart!
Or to savagely attack and slash
With sharpened sword!
Or to battle with blunt instrument
Hacking—striking—pounding!
I would slaughter this unseen enemy
By stoning, bruising bone and flesh!
Or, cursing and screaming,
I would intimidate in rage of sound!
Let me fight this dread, dark thing.

After violent thoughts dissipate,
My best fight is fought
By simply lying still to follow
Prescribed course of radiation
At oncology treatment center,
Though I would rather forget the fray
And go running outdoors to play.

They "Light Up My Life"
I'm zapped by radiation once a day,
So when I'm dressed and start to dash away,
I quite expect each passerby to say,
"You look just simply radiant today."

Response to a Get-well Card
Your note was heartening.
So good of you to be a part
of helping in my need.
Just to let you know
that healing is happening.
My tribulation was not the end,
but a strange form of beginning.
So here's to walking a little longer
in the world with you, my friend.

Following the Storm
Then,
peeping around the corner
of personal despair
there comes that fey fairy,
Hope!

After Life
It used to be
that theaters would show
a short-reel cartoon
where Bugs Bunny
would always outwit
Elmer Fudd and win,
before the final words
THE END.

It was only then
that the wide-screen,
technicolor
main feature could begin.

Cancer
As with roulette,
in this hideous
new game of chance
players are chosen
by wherever
the next lump lands.

Like a giant numbered wheel
without rule or plan,
my mind spins.
Why play this
insidious game
when no one wins?

Ninety-Percent Winner
In this competitive world
one hundred percent
is the most you can expect.

I have just been assured
of only ninety percent
chance of long life.
Yet I am content to celebrate
over whatever I can get,
for with this disease
there are no guarantees.

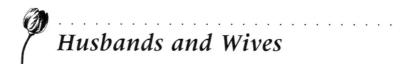

Husbands and Wives

Breast cancer is a very personal disease that affects a woman's body and sense of self in intimate ways. It also affects those she loves. Support from loved ones is one of the most important tools a woman has to cope with cancer. The husbands who wrote the stories in this chapter offered support through many ways: listening, humor, planned activities, back rubs, housework, and child care. And love, most importantly, love.

"Advice for the Cancer-lorn" offers concrete suggestions for handling surgery and the postoperative period. "To Love, Honor, and Listen" discusses one husband's role as sounding board as his wife comes to terms with the diagnosis.

"On Life's Trade-offs" talks about the long-term adjustments to having had two different kinds of cancer. "Second Pair $1" shows how humor can help us get through the worst of times.

"Even Doctors Get Breast Cancer" and "An Alternative Form of Early Detection" illustrate that professional knowledge may make the tough decisions easier to understand but not easier to accept.

The subject of hereditary cancer is the background in "All in the Family, parts 1 and 2," as members of one woman's family, as well as her husband's mother, had died of cancer.

Advice for the Cancer-lorn

Susan Cambigue-Tracey

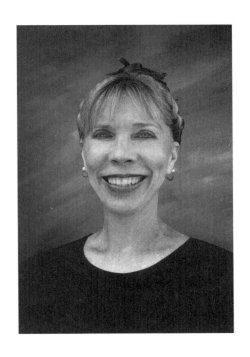

Susan has been a dancer and dance educator for thirty-five years. She has a degree in physical education/dance, but today draws upon the experiential education she has acquired from her travels throughout the United States as a Dance/Movement Specialist for the National Endowment for the Arts' "Artists in Schools" program. Susan has been chosen for residencies, workshops, and performances in Germany and Africa. For seven years she was the Artistic Director for the Free Flight Improvisational Dance Company; for fifteen years she has been an Arts Education Consultant with The Performing Tree, the Music Center Education Division, and the Galef Institute. She has been President of the California Dance Educators Association, teaches part time at Loyola Marymount University, is Chair Elect of the California Alliance for Arts Education, and is currently Director of Public Affairs for the Los Angeles Music Center Education Division.

Medical Bio

In December 1987, when Susan was forty-seven years old, a routine screening mammogram demonstrated the presence of microcalcifications in her right breast. At that time, she was experiencing no breast symptoms, and the recommendation for biopsy was based upon her mammographic findings. In mid-December, she had a biopsy that demonstrated extensive intraductal breast cancer. There was no pathologic evidence that the breast cancer had invaded the tissue surrounding the milk ducts.

After consultation with her surgeon, Susan made the decision to proceed with a right modified radical mastectomy a few days after Christmas. She made an uneventful recovery from her surgery and at this point has not had breast reconstruction. She is well and without evidence of recurrent breast cancer.

It was the day after my biopsy. I was back at work, trying to complete several projects before the Christmas holiday. The phone rang, and my doctor spoke sadly but with authority: "I am afraid I have bad news for you. Please come to my office right away." I drove to the meeting with a sense of urgency and disbelief.

"We found cancer. You have a few choices, but I recommend a modified radical mastectomy for your right breast. If we act quickly, your prognosis is very bright and you may be able to avoid radiation and chemotherapy."

My stomach contracted into a tight knot, and blood raced through my arteries, creating a feeling of panic. Unreality enveloped me. My doctor knew this and guided me through the briefing with clinical professionalism and compassion. "Those are your options. The choice is up to you, and I will respect any choice you make." I left his office, inwardly vibrating with impulses of flight and fright but forcing myself to make a contained and outwardly pleasant departure.

. . . .
Coming to terms with cancer

How can this be happening to me? Why me? There must be a mistake! They got my biopsy slides mixed up with someone else's. I won't let them do it. There MUST be another solution. What did I do wrong? I don't deserve this. I'll just leave this office and won't come back. They can't make me have an operation.

It is unthinkable to lose my breast. I fold my arms protectively about myself as the cold air contracts my skin and raises goose bumps in waves throughout my body. I hold my right breast in the car, making sure it is still there.

What will my family think? It will destroy my parents. My mother had a mastectomy a few years ago and didn't tell me until it was all over. Did she feel this way? Was she embarrassed and humiliated? How did she survive the chemotherapy and radiation? I wasn't even there to support her. She wanted it to be a private affair. She has never discussed her health with me.

Only my father stood by her side, but they are a very private couple, and I respect that.

This is a disease that I can't even see. I HAVE CANCER! I can't stand it. I'll kill myself. I'll leave town. I'll say goodbye to everyone. I'll write them a note, then go away to another city and live my life out. If I die, I die. At least no one will be hurt if I leave now. My God, I could die!

Several colonies of cancer cells are living and reproducing in my right breast. They could travel by bloodstream and settle elsewhere. I feel afraid. I feel panicky. I feel helpless. I feel a deep and overwhelming grief about the possibility of losing my breast. I have had breasts since I was ten years old. They have been an integral part of me for thirty-seven years. Even though I was still a child when they appeared, they announced to the world that I had attained the status of womanhood. At first, I hated them for the attention they drew to me, but they were a symbol of my femininity, and I grew to love their curving effect on my body. It became clear to me, as these memories stimulated my senses, that no one was going to take my breast.

Maybe this problem will go away by itself. I will visualize it disappearing. I am very strong, very spiritually oriented. I am conscious of eating right and maintaining my health. I am a dancer; my body is my instrument of self-expression. It obeys me. I can, and have, overcome pain and other physical limitations. I will conquer this. I will do it alone.

I must get out of here. Where can I hide? Nowhere! It's useless. Oh, what the hell, I'll just tell them to take my breast. Take both of them. I don't care anymore. Operate. Get it over with. Put me to sleep and don't tell me what you're going to do. Maybe I won't even wake up.

Paul will be shocked. He'll retreat into himself and go on as if nothing is wrong. He will never be able to deal with this. He'll still love me, but he won't be able to find me attractive. He has always loved my breasts. How can we ever make love again?

Okay, get hold of yourself. You've had to handle problems before. First, you recovered from a divorce. You learned things about yourself and developed into a wiser, more aware person. Then, you had to survive the death of Julie, the daughter you cherished and adored. When her future evaporated, you lived through the grief. At nineteen years old, she stood on the edge of life with her golden wings spread wide. You watched her tumble into the sea like Icarus, the child of Daedalus. You found the strength to go on. People say that bad things only happen to those who are strong enough to handle them; on the contrary, I feel that tragedies force you to become strong enough to survive.

This is like death, too. Your body will be changed, but will YOU be changed? In every tragedy, there are lessons to be learned, new insights to be seen, hidden strengths to be exercised. Even the ordinary person has the opportunity to be extraordinary by displaying dignity and courage in the face of fear—and you have never considered yourself ordinary.

Can I be helped? Can surgery really handle this terrible problem? Can I return to a normal life? Will people relate to me differently? Will they become afraid that they will catch what I have? Will I respond differently to them? Will I be able to face friends? Will I be able to face myself?

I absorb what the doctor has told me. I don't like him very much at this moment. It is his fault. He found the cancer and made it real to me. As I looked at him in stunned horror, he said, "By operating and removing the entire breast, we can save your life. You can look forward to many more years of zestful living and loving."

I ask myself, "Why is he talking this way to me?" This must be a joke. It's more than that, it's a plot! It reminds me of a movie I once saw where people conspired to drive a woman insane by telling her lies. I feel so healthy now, not even slightly ill. I look healthy. I feel vibrant and alive. I dance, teach, and write with power and concentration. If I have this operation, I won't feel this well for several weeks, maybe months. And what about my dancing? Will it affect the way I can move? I've heard that it will be difficult to have full range of movement in my arm after the lymph nodes are removed. My doctor says I will return to normal and be even better off than before, because I won't have this terrible disease threatening me. Can I believe him?

My gynecologist calls to give me moral support. He is kind and empathetic but says I must act quickly. He recommends that I get a second opinion, so I go to the Comprehensive Cancer Center. As I sit waiting for my appointment, I see people who are in different stages of cancer: several children are bald from continuous radiation treatments; a young boy with tubes attached to his arm is lying on a couch, weakened by chemotherapy; a baby, born with cancer, sobs in his mother's arms; a young man, thin and scarred, stares into space. These glimpses at the ravages of cancer not caught in time unnerve and depress me.

Then a handsome, jolly Santa enters the room, filling us with warm smiles. He tenderly approaches each child with a supportive remark, a hearty laugh, and a candy cane. I try to avoid catching his eye, but he comes directly to me and says, "You look like you need a candy cane too." I later learned he was a patient, dying of cancer, who had long ago lost his hair and had many scars from a multitude of operations. He certainly wasn't lamenting life. I felt both inspired by his attitude and ashamed of my own self-pity.

The doctor I am to see, a young and beautiful woman, greets me and discusses my case. Her advice is basically the same as my doctor's. When I bring up the subject of alternative treatments, she encourages me to find out all I can but not to risk my chances for the complete and immediate recovery that surgery would almost certainly assure.

I feel sure that she and my doctor must be conspiring against me. She is supporting his evil strategy to maim me. I'll get a third opinion. With the help of my doctor's nurse, I get my mammogram results and biopsy slides from the pathology department. Armed with these, I trot off to UCLA and the Bowyer Clinic. The third and fourth doctors give me the same diagnosis and the same advice. Now there are four doctors telling me that I must rid my body of the invading mass of killer cells. They all encourage me to be strong, to make the optimum choice for my life.

My husband knows. I tell him in clinical verbiage and professional tones, passing on the information as if I had pressed the *play* button to a medical cassette. Then I break down and cry like a child, wanting him to protect me, to change everything, to make it go away. I suggest that we just forget it all and go around the world together. He looks at me tenderly, letting me babble and spill out fantasy solutions to this real problem.

I challenge him by asking what he thinks I should do. He says, "Well, I can't tell you what to do. It is, after all, your life. But I would like to share it with you for as long as possible. If you decide to have the operation, at least it's a decorative part they would be removing, one that you can do without. It would be much worse for a dancer to lose her foot or arm."

I think of my friend Marianne Quirk, a dancer who did lose her arm. She had the courage to get a prosthesis and the imagination to continue to dance and choreograph. My problem starts to seem so small in comparison. But I still worry about how I'll look in a leotard. I begin to think beyond the surgery, toward reconstruction. I am aware of how lucky I am to live in a time of advanced medical possibilities.

I continue to wrestle with indecision for several days. The doctors are patient and understanding but urge me to face the factor of time. Each day I wait, I become more vulnerable. I talk to friends. I read as much as I can about cancer. I investigate alternative choices. I pray. I go to my church and get some counseling. I write down the pros and cons of the limited choices I have.

I think about my breasts and how they have served me. They have allowed me to nurse my two children. During their childhood, Julie and Heather gained comfort from them, pressing against me in spontaneous gestures of love and burying their heads between them during times of stress. My breasts have provided sensuous moments of pleasure for both my husband and me. They have decorated my form and identified me with universal womanhood.

I begin to realize that it is time to say good-bye to this intimate part of myself. The breast has become a time capsule ready to explode into millions of destructive colonists, raping my territory. I must find the courage to move through this problem. I realize that I cannot stand still and wait for imminent disaster.

My breast will be sacrificed in exchange for life. My breast has harbored grief, fear, anger, and love. I begin to perceive that the shattering events in my life have manifested themselves in the form of cancer. My daughter's death left me in a place of such sorrow that I no longer fully valued my own life. She was an extension of myself and represented my future, as well as her own. I need to take back the responsibility of creating my own happiness and release her from that burden.

The shock of understanding that I am now in a life-threatening situation is like a glass of ice water being thrown in my face. Unlike my daughter, who died in an automobile accident, I have the choice of whether to shorten or extend my life. This realization lifts me out of my apathy. I know now that I want to live. I want to enjoy more fully the people who are in my life. I want to make my life count by contributing more of myself. I have been somewhat on hold for three years. Most people think I am functioning well, but it is cancer that makes me see how much energy is being trapped by my grief.

So I did make the choice to have a modified radical mastectomy of my right breast. It is hard to believe, but I have been exuberant since the morning after surgery. I feel that I have been given a new chance at life. I have more things I want to do, more love I want to give, and more joy I want to express.

Yes, it was a shock to see my chest without a breast, to confront my ribs, which suddenly stood out prominently. It was hard to accept the scar that marks this passage in my life. But my wise and loving husband said, "Now you can claim to be a descendant of the legendary Amazon women. They were said to be courageous, beautiful, and strong. They had the right breast removed in order to shoot their arrows more precisely toward their target. Perhaps now that yours is gone, you can do the same."

. . . .

Things I found helpful before and after breast surgery

Preparation for surgery

1. Take the time to get a second opinion. Read about cancer and find out what you can and cannot control about your own case. I found out all that I could so that when I made the decision to have the recommended mastectomy, I was certain about it.

2. Begin to handle your feelings of shock, grief, anger, and loss by fully expressing them to yourself and to your partner, family members, and friends.

Cry and let the natural healing process begin with an acceptance of your situation.

3. If possible, plan a lovely evening for yourself the night before surgery. Make it happy and full of things you enjoy (a good meal, a fire, a romantic interlude, a movie, a play, a piece of fudge, etc.).

4. Make a plan for yourself. This helps you get back in control of your life. Make a list of things you could easily do during recovery. I found that I could resume old projects, start new ones, catch up on my reading, listen to tapes, write to neglected friends, complete a sweater I began two years ago. It gave me things to look forward to and made me feel productive.

5. Pack a small bag for the hospital. Include a toothbrush, toothpaste, brush or comb, two nightgowns, perhaps a light robe, and socks or slippers to keep your feet warm. I also took a fragrant soap, some makeup, my Walkman and a few favorite tapes, two pairs of clean panties, some tampons (I always get my period during a crisis), a book of short stories, a trashy novel, a package of gum, and a small package of M&M's. I can deal with anything if I have a package of M&M's! Everything else is provided for you, but do be sure you have clothing—including a comfortable and large sweater or blouse—to wear home.

6. My husband and I decided to take some photographs of me before the surgery. At first I was hesitant about how this would make me feel, but the photos turned out well, and I feel very pleased to have them now. The photos remind me that I can look this way again if I decide to have reconstruction.

7. The assistant to your surgeon will answer your questions and give you needed moral support. Ask for information on support groups in your area. Take advantage of this help. I did, and it made a huge difference!

In the hospital after surgery

1. When you are aware enough to see where you are after waking from the anesthetic, begin to look around the room and notice specific objects within your range of view. Observe things that are near and far, things that are large and small. This will help bring you back into the here and now. Drugs can make you feel confused. It helps to get back in control of time, space, and energy.

2. As soon as possible after surgery, get up and brush your teeth, wash your face, put a little makeup on, and change into one of your own nightgowns. It does wonders for your spirits.

3. When the nurse gives you the go-ahead, get up and walk around your room or around the ward. You'll probably want to go to the bathroom. I encouraged myself to walk around the ward a few times each day. I always felt better because my system got stimulated; I even rested better afterward. If

you get sick and vomit, just use the little tray the hospital provides and feel happy that your body is working to rid your system of the drugs used in surgery. Trust your body to know what to do—and this advice comes from someone who hates to vomit. It did make me feel much better.

4. If you want a wonderful and healthful treat, make arrangements ahead of time for a professional masseuse to come to the hospital on one of the days following your surgery. Ask him/her to massage your feet, hands, shoulders, neck, and head. This can be done easily in your hospital bed, and it assists in the healing process by increasing circulation, relaxing you, and stimulating all your systems. The cost will not be covered by your insurance, but it is well worth it. I had a terrible headache after my surgery, and the massage helped.

5. Ask your doctor about supplemental vitamins and minerals that assist specific types of healing. For my mastectomy, I supplemented with the following:

- Vitamin E, to assist with healing scars;
- Arnica, a homeopathic remedy that assists with healing;
- SeroLymph Forto, to assist with the healing and strengthening of the lymph nodes;
- Vitamin B Complex, for general strength and energy.

6. Decide that you can heal easily. Think positive thoughts about yourself. If it appeals to you, keep a journal, or record your thoughts on a tape recorder. Listen to your needs and find ways to respond to them. Don't be afraid to ask for help. Most friends would like to know specifically how to help you. They like to be trusted and needed by you; it makes them feel worthwhile and valued. The great philosopher Kahlil Gibran wrote in *The Prophet:* "And you receivers—and you are all receivers—assume no weight of gratitude, lest you lay a yoke upon yourself and upon him who gives. Rather rise together with the giver on his gifts as on wings."

During recovery

1. Pamper yourself. Get others to pamper you too. Let people help you, but only those you want near you and who flow positive, healing energy to you and wish you well.

2. Keep your spirits up. Yes, you may fall into periods of sadness or depression, but you have the power to lift yourself out. You are alive, and there are many people with more difficult problems than yours to deal with. It helps to think of ten problems worse than yours. Yours will begin to reduce in time.

3. Take a short walk each day, preferably outside. Notice the wonderful things that you may not have taken the time to see in a while. Nature

will seem even more creative and wondrous. Your ability to observe, appreciate, and participate in life will bring you great joy, if you let it.

4. If you can't wash your hair, have someone assist you or drive you to the beauty shop. I found it well worth the effort. It felt so good to have my hair fresh and clean.

5. Every morning, try to brush your teeth, wash your face, comb your hair, and, if you wish, put on a little makeup. When I look better, I can usually fool myself into thinking that I feel better.

6. Change from your nightclothes into some loose clothing for the day, even if you are in bed or resting much of the time. It can perk you up and make you feel that you are in the well group.

7. Try to visualize what you will look like when your bandages are removed. Prepare yourself. Ask the doctor what the scars will look like and how long they will take to heal. The more information you have, the better prepared you can be for the shock of losing one or both breasts.

8. Help your mate, family, or friends confront the scars, if this is appropriate. My husband is very squeamish and faints at the mention of blood. First, I confronted the bandages and the fact that my chest was flat. There was nothing there—very hard to believe. Then, I asked my husband to just look at the bandages. We did this quietly and slowly. I encouraged him to verbalize his feelings. He thought that I looked weird and unnatural. I just let him absorb the change.

Next, I took off the temporary gauze bandages after the doctor told me I could. I took my first shower, and then I called my husband in again. I asked if he thought he could look at the scar so that we could both begin to accept the change and not let it be a barrier between us. He reluctantly agreed. I had covered myself with a towel. He asked me to move the towel across my chest, a half-inch at a time, until I was completely exposed. His first reaction was that I looked like I belonged in a Frankenstein movie. I thought so too. Together we commented on how weird it looked and how ugly it was—and it was! We got more descriptive and more enthusiastic about describing it, and then we began to laugh. Did I ever imagine I would not have breasts? No! Well, here I am without one. We repeated this drama for the next few days until it became rather boring.

This step can be done in many different ways. You need to find your own way of handling it. But do handle it, and do it as soon as possible. You will find the strength within yourself to deal with it, and a huge weight will be taken from your shoulders. Courage!

9. Contact Reach to Recovery. This organization is wonderful and very responsive to your needs. It will find people who have been through a

similar experience and who have survived in good condition. My husband called and talked about his fears and feelings with another husband. He said he gained new understanding and felt much better. Volunteers will visit you in the hospital or at home and take you through the entire process, step by step. They will also tell you about reconstruction and help you get fitted for a prosthesis. The better department stores also have trained people who can assist you in getting fitted for one or two prostheses. But I have tried another way: making my own. I have made several and rotate their use.

Recipe for a Birdseed Breast: Start with a knee-high nylon stocking (your choice of natural colors). Pour birdseed into the toe. Experiment by placing it inside your bra and molding it until the amount seems to match the breast that remains. Pack it loosely. Tie the nylon stocking firmly and cut it off close to the knot. The knot looks just like a nipple when turned outward inside your bra. The big surprise is that it looks very natural, is inexpensive, and feels extremely comfortable.

10. Keep your sense of humor. There are things you can find to laugh about. Focus on them. It releases anxiety and lightens the situation.

11. Though we don't put in requests for them, difficult challenges can help us find new insight into ourselves and others. I discovered I liked myself just as well without my right breast. It certainly changed my lifestyle temporarily, but I also had time to think, relax, and find new interests. I depend upon my body and value how it looks and moves since I am a dancer and teacher. In just a few weeks, I will be able to go back to my normal routine, for I was able to avoid chemotherapy and radiation treatments. If you need to go through this next phase, perhaps you can add your thoughts to mine and assist someone else through this process. We all need to support each other.

Exercises for postmastectomy

It was very important for me to get my arms moving with full range again. The following are exercises that I found very helpful.

It is important to work slowly and with an easy, stretching motion. Bouncing or forcing the range of your movement by using strong, quick, or forceful actions can injure you. Breathe deeply and slowly as you work, letting the breath relax your muscles enough to stretch easily and without injury. Stretching is a slow process, and your range increases with repetition and by slowly sustaining the stretch. I found that music made the daily process more enjoyable and successful. Select music that is relaxing.

For the first week, work for about 5 minutes at a time, several times a day. The second week, increase your concentration and endurance to 10 or 15 minutes, adding a few general body stretches, as well. The third week, try to be consistent and don't stop just because you are feeling so much better. Keep repeating these exercises until you have full range and strength of movement. Don't settle for less!

1. Standing or sitting: Curve your arms in front of your torso, below your waist. Breathe in and slowly raise them upward, keeping the curved shape in both arms. Breathe out fully and evenly as you lower your arms, following the same path. Repeat this movement sequence several times. Hold your stomach in and lengthen your lower back muscles as you do this. As you move your arms, lower your shoulder blades to keep tension out of your shoulders.

2. Standing or sitting: Place your arms at the side of your torso. Turn your palms toward the front. Press your arms and hands downward and as you continue pressing down and out, lift them away from the sides of your torso, continuing upward with a continuous flow of energy. Slowly bring your arms and hands down. As you do this, be aware of pulling your shoulder blades downward, contracting your stomach muscles, and lengthening the lower back.

3. Standing or sitting: With your arms bent and hands touching the shoulders, slowly circle your elbows as fully as possible in one direction. Do this several times and then circle them in the opposite direction.

4. Standing or sitting: Reach your arms out to the sides and slowly move them together to cross your torso in a hugging position (arms across chest). Slowly unfold them until your arms are again wide and out to the sides. Work to increase the range of movement. When you begin to feel some success, lift your elbows while in the "hugging" position. This will begin to make it possible for you to put sweaters on by yourself.

5. Standing or sitting: Clasp your hands together with laced fingers pointing toward your chin. Hold them at waist height, with elbows out as wide as possible. Pressing your hands together, move them upward, drawing a straight line up the center of your body. Keep them as close as possible to your chest, chin, nose, and forehead. Go as far as you can, using your breath to assist you. Take a deep breath in before you begin and move your arms and hands upward as you slowly and deeply breathe out. Repeat this as you continue upward.

6. Standing: Lean forward with a straight back, and place your hands on your knees. As you do this, bend your knees slightly and keep your elbows straight. Breathe in fully. As you breathe out, take four slow counts to round your back, beginning the action at your tailbone and extending it to include your neck and head. Take another full breath in and begin to arch your spine as you breathe out. Make sure that you begin the action at your tailbone

and continue it up the spine until you complete it by arching your neck and head. Repeat these two actions several times to warm up and extend the range of motion in your spine. (This exercise also involves your rib cage and chest and is a good one to continue throughout your life.)

7. Standing or sitting: Put on some music and move your arms slowly and with a feeling of strength and beauty in movements of your own choice. Think of exploring these possibilities: full circles and half circles, opening and closing gestures, arms moving together and separately, directions of up and down, side to side, diagonally across the body. Try twisting, curving, or turning the torso with the arm motions and adding the head and spine to start or extend the arm movements.

8. Standing or sitting: After a couple of weeks of doing the other exercises, place your hands on the tops of your shoulders. Work slowly to lift your elbows so they are at the same level as your shoulders. Do this several times, working to stretch higher each time.

9. Daily activities: Use your arms as much as possible during your recovery by combing your hair, washing your hair, reaching for things that require some extra effort or stretch, and sweeping the floor (not easy at first).

To Love, Honor, and Listen

Paul Tracey (Susan's husband)

If you think about a bad thing happening, well, you might make it happen. So you don't say anything. But you do think it. You can't help thinking it, knowing the statistics.

I thought about it every time Susan went for a regular checkup, and I breathed a great sigh of relief every time she came home with a clean report. But I did worry about her breast. Why did it hurt so often? That seemed unnatural. But if she kept going for regular checkups the way she did so faithfully, I supposed there was nothing to worry about.

But this time her doctor got suspicious and asked for a biopsy. The thought of that alone almost laid me out on the floor. I do that very easily. Once my daughter ran through a plate-glass window and cut the back of her leg with a long shard of glass, and blood spurted out. I was all right until she asked me to come into the emergency room with her to hold her hand. I did precisely as she asked, and when the doctor came in, there I was, still holding her hand, but lying on the floor!

I got through the first operation very well, controlling my outrage that some strange person would be cutting up my wife and that she would willingly let him do it. I didn't really want to know much about it, but part of the job of being husband to Susan is listening. I suppose it was my own fault; that was one of the promises I made to her at our wedding: "I promise to listen." Sounded good at the time.

But I was very cheered by the surgeon's report that things looked good. Unfortunately, the lab report was not so good. Poor Susan rushed off to hear the worst news—she had cancer. What were her choices? None, really. I had always been led to believe that if you catch cancer early, you can do something about it. I did not realize that "doing something" meant removing the whole breast! That's the way it was in our case. Wasn't that rather violent? Biblical, no less: "If thy breast offend thee, cut it off!"

Of course, I knew right away what had to be done. I heard the choices; all of them were chancy at best. And even the radical surgery could not guarantee that the cancer would be caught. So we had to make up our minds in a hurry before the damn thing spread any further. My heart sank when Susan came out so vehemently against the only possible choice.

My first wife died in a car accident. We lost our eldest daughter in another accident. That's unlucky, to say the least. But now, if Susan insisted on dying by not making the obvious choice, people would think that I was simply careless! I make light of things; that's how I deal with life. But in the familiar spot in the pit of my stomach there came that wretched feeling again. Am I going to suffer another loss?

Luckily, Susan has a good head on her shoulders and determination to match. You have never seen anyone research an issue with such single-mindedness—the books, the second opinions, the third and fourth opinions, the rushing about town to meet with doctors here and there. Every single doctor took a look at the offending breast and gave it a poke. Why? In her case, there wasn't even a lump. You couldn't SEE anything wrong, and there was nothing to feel. We had to rely on the word of the experts. Strange thoughts invade your mind . . . could ALL the doctors be in a giant plot together? Did each call ahead to tell the next doctor we were coming? Paranoia!

But we worked hard together, reassured each other, made absolutely certain that we had done everything humanly possible. We wanted to make sure that we would never have to say, "If only we had done this, or that, or the other." And then we decided. She decided, really; it had to come from her. I tried not to tell her what to do, but I'm sure she knew what I thought. It would be easier if it was her idea.

Once the decision was made to go ahead with the surgery, the agonizing was over. We knew there would be agony ahead, but at least we were clear as to our direction. I called the Reach to Recovery people in Santa Monica, and they connected me with someone who had been through the same thing. I was reassured that my thoughts were on the right track. I know that a breast is more than just a pound of flesh. It represents so much more, femininity itself. Obviously, I had to make sure that Susan knew I would find her equally as attractive after the operation as before.

And then the day came. We woke up at 4:30 A.M. so that Susan could take herself through a dance routine! Can you imagine living with someone like that? She wanted to be in tip-top condition before the operation. You have to admire someone like that. You admire them bleary-eyed. At 6:30 A.M. we arrived at the hospital, and I took several walks along the corridors. We had never talked about making out a will, but I bet I wasn't the only one who thought about it at that time.

Thank God for my friend Jamil. He stood by me, keeping my mind off the operation by playing Scrabble. Then the surgeon came in and told us how well it went and what great chest muscles she had. All right, but I wish I hadn't had to imagine how he had seen them . . . from the inside! Susan took a terribly long time to regain consciousness, three hours instead of one.

Then the recovery, the toughness of this woman who would not allow herself a minute of luxury to be an invalid. She had to be up and walking around the ward long before anyone thought it was advisable.

We went home, and the bandages were so huge that I did not yet see that she was flat on one side. This was a moment of reprieve, because when the bandages did finally come off, it was a shock—a real shock, even after all the preparations, the counseling, the visual images I had conjured up. There was simply nothing there. It was flatter than a man's chest. The join was a curious one. Two different sorts of skin were drawn together: the suntanned cleavage skin and the pale belly skin. I could not help but recall the look of Frankenstein's monster, the stitches were so huge. I looked at it for a long time, not because I wanted to but because Susan had this crazy idea that I had to face it. Perhaps she was right, but I confronted it sitting on the bed, ready to lie flat if necessary!

Then came the phone calls. I could not imagine how some people got the news, but it spread like the plague. Outside of a few close friends, I really didn't want everyone to know, to have to suffer along with us. We wanted to spare them the agony and the fear that they might also have this affliction, which was especially scary because of the lack of any lump. But they did find out; practically everyone is a blabbermouth when it comes to this! And the ones who called were upset because we hadn't told them. It was hard to explain that we were trying to do them a favor.

So that was it—phase one. Reconstruction is the next decision to be made, and you can be sure that it will be well researched before we go ahead. Meanwhile, Susan and I love each other even more than before, having been reminded once again just how fragile life can be. (P.S. Thank you, God, but we don't need to be reminded anymore!)

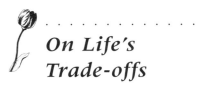

On Life's Trade-offs

Vicki Gillespie Mickelsen

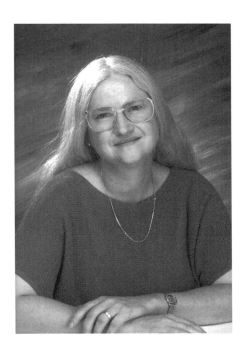

Vicki lives in a 100-year-old house, which she and her husband, David, have lovingly restored, and she recently spearheaded a movement to have her neighborhood declared a historic district. She also loves singing Renaissance music, collecting textiles and books, and living in foreign countries. Vicki has been married to David since 1967; they have two daughters. She has a Ph.D. in Spanish and taught Spanish at a local university for five years and also taught English as a Second Language in the United States and Africa. She is currently the managing editor of the documentation department of a medical software company. She manages a staff of twelve writers, so, as she puts it, she's still "teaching," with the additional pleasure of creating beautiful books. She also works as a freelance writer. Vicki has steadfastly and patiently served as one of the editors of this book.

Medical Bio

In the fall of 1974, Vicki was diagnosed as having nodular sclerosing Hodgkin's disease, a cancer of the lymph nodes. She went through radiation therapy for the treatment of this problem and has never had any evidence of recurrence. The radiation treatment that rendered her cured of the Hodgkin's disease did expose her breast tissue to significant levels of radiation.

In August of 1987, Vicki first noted a yellowish nipple discharge from her right breast. She was evaluated for this problem in November of the same year, and very asymmetrical mammographic findings were identified. The recommended biopsy of the involved nipple duct identified a diffuse intraductal cancer of the right breast. Vicki underwent a right modified radical mastectomy with immediate prosthetic reconstruction. There was no evidence of any metastatic cancer in her axillary lymph nodes. Vicki has had one procedure to revise her reconstruction result and, at this time, is without any evidence of recurrent breast cancer.

There are moments when your life changes forever. It's 1974. I'm thirty years old and expecting our first child. We're sitting in the oncologist's office after the lump I found on my neck has been biopsied. He says something like, "I have some bad news and some good news. The bad news is, you have Hodgkin's disease, a type of cancer of the lymph system; the good news is, the cure rate now is around 90 percent." There's every hope in the world for me—none for the baby.

For months after that, I live in an emotional deep freeze. I do what I am told by a battery of competent and caring physicians, supported by husband, family, and friends. I have an abortion; I have radiation on my chest; I have a staging laparotomy to biopsy the liver, lymph nodes, and bone marrow, and remove the spleen; I have more radiation on my stomach and back. Finally, six months later, I emerge from daily trips to the hospital and go on with my life.

Gradually, the deep freeze eases. The hard core of grief for the baby is buried. I adjust to being a "cancer victim" and make bad jokes about it. After two years, I'm officially declared "in remission," and life finds a new normal.

Fourteen years and two kids later, I'm sitting across from the same surgeon who did the laparotomy; he's now a specialist in breast care. "Now, really," I say, "we have to stop meeting like this." I'm there because of a mysterious discharge from the right breast; the mammogram looked normal, but antibiotics did not clear it up. He says, "it's probably not cancer, but let's do a biopsy to be sure." Well, it is.

What I have is comedocarcinoma, growing in the milk glands. There is no lump; only a marked difference between right and left breast mammograms made him suspect something odd. It is a very slow-growing type; I may have had it for several years. And the real irony of the situation—it's probably a result of the radiation therapy received for the Hodgkin's disease.

Well, I'm willing to trade a breast for those fourteen years and two kids.

....

The second time around

I had thought a lot in the intervening years about how I handled my fear and grief the first time, and this time I did it differently. I protested. I asked lots of questions. I looked for alternatives. I complained. I talked to my therapist, my friends, and my husband about what I was feeling. I let them, especially my husband, support and comfort me, instead of stiff-upper-lipping it alone. And when I agreed to the mastectomy, I felt that it was my choice, not some horrible reality thrust upon me against my will.

Instead of freezing emotionally, I cried. Occasionally I panicked. When I had Hodgkin's, I was so grief-stricken about the baby, I didn't care if I lived or not. This time I did. Once, shopping for Christmas presents in a kitchenware store, I looked at all the lovely things I might never own, looked at my lovely daughters I might not see grow up, and I started to shake. From somewhere, words of comfort came to me: "Well, even if you die, it won't be today, so don't worry about it." Epiphany among the garlic presses.

During the time between the diagnosis and the mastectomy, I learned all I could about the disease and the treatments. I talked to people who have had breast cancer and heard about their experiences. And, as I always do when troubled, I went to my favorite bookstore, trusting that the wisdom I needed would serendipitously present itself. In this case, I found a book called *Love, Medicine, and Miracles* by Dr. Bernie Siegel.

In the last several years, his books have become quite famous, but at this time, the first one had just come out. His optimism and approach were exactly what I needed in order to feel that I had some control over my reactions to the disease and the treatment, if not over the disease itself. His exercises, and those of the Simontons in *Getting Well Again*, were close to a kind of meditation I was already practicing, so I felt comfortable with their advice and found it very helpful.

The most difficult situation I faced in this first period was being put in the position of comforting and supporting my friends who were upset about my having cancer. It's as if some people are so afraid of cancer that they immediately project their own emotions onto your situation and can't cope with it. So they turn to you for comfort (well, after all, you're the expert). But I needed all my resources for myself and my family during this time; I learned to stay away from the people who drained me emotionally and to rely on those who could handle their own fears as well as help me with mine.

....
All I want for Christmas is a new right breast

The surgery took place on December 18. It was about what I expected, although the doctor felt that our request to have the breast stuffed for the mantelpiece was not one he could fulfill. Since I work for a company that makes software for hospitals, I spent my time before surgery quizzing the nurses about their software and how they liked it, rather than worrying about the operation. It also helped to have a caring and supportive surgical team, family, and hospital staff. I always felt that I was well looked after and well informed about hospital procedures and what to expect. Still, there is always a moment of truth when the needle goes in, a brief prayer that I will wake up again.

The hospital stay was also uneventful, at least as I remember it now. I slept a lot, walked a bit more each day, entertained family and visitors, read, listened to music, spent a lot of time figuring out how to turn over and to get out of and into bed. There was a period of what I called "crazy pain" when the muscles in my chest seemed to go haywire, but I learned to avoid the movements that would trigger it.

I came home a couple of days before Christmas. My mother-in-law and sister-in-law were with us, so I was really pampered. They were amazed and appalled when I went Christmas shopping the third day I was home, but I felt like seeing if I could handle a trip out into the real world after being cloistered in the hospital.

All through this period, I felt we were all coping well. We were cheerful, made jokes, played with the kids, wrapped presents, and tried to live normally. However, I realized how very worried we had been when we finally got the word that the bone scan had come back negative and the lymph nodes were clean. I cried from relief. I cried again when the tumor board decided that I did not need further treatment, either chemotherapy or radiation. This was especially important because I had already received my maximum lifetime dosage of radiation and any more would put me at risk of developing other, even less desirable, forms of cancer.

The week after Christmas, David and I went to buy a new breast. I had chosen reconstruction and had received a temporary implant that would gradually be expanded with weekly injections of saline solution. But full expansion was months away, and since I am rather well-endowed, I felt that my lopsided condition would be too visible. So we bought a prosthesis. The experience was one in which humor very nearly failed me. I went through the motions, all the time shrieking *no no no* inside. I don't know if the prosthesis made the experience of losing a breast too real to handle, or if it was somehow too blatant a denial of that reality. In any case, I rarely wore it. My four year old, however, was enchanted by it. She fondled it, cooed at it, and ended up wearing it on her head.

. . . .
Life in the lopsided lane

Although surgery is a grim way to spend Christmas, there were advantages. The kids were distracted, my friends had time to visit, and I didn't miss any work. On January 2, I clambered into the car, figured out how to shift with my left hand, and headed off to the office. My boss and coworkers were concerned but not overprotective. We had a book to get to the printer, so no one had time to sit around and worry about me. About a month later, I was sent to work on-site at the company we were writing software manuals for. Since I was faced with a host of strangers, I would set out each morning with the fake breast in place. But by midafternoon, it would be hidden in the desk drawer. Then I quit wearing it altogether. I learned that most people don't seem to see the imbalance. For a while, I thought they were being polite, but I have since discovered that even the people I work with most closely never suspected I had had breast cancer until I told them.

They would have known, however, if they had been watching a local TV channel in February, when David and I appeared with our doctor and some other patients to share our experience and answer questions from viewers. I realized from the questions how uninformed most people are about the disease and treatments, and how this ignorance makes it seem even more scary than it is.

We did go through the implant process. I say *we* because for a while, David valiantly strove to insert the needle into the little tube and deposit the week's portion of saline solution. But he wasn't fond of the process, and he was glad when we had the doctor do it instead. In May, the temporary was replaced by a permanent implant in yet another operation. This time I elected to have local anesthetic and was very pleased with the ease of recovery.

I was not pleased with the results, however. Even though the implant is as large as it can be, I am still very lopsided. Because I grew up during the era of Marilyn and Jayne and turned out to resemble them in that salient characteristic, I have always considered my breasts to be one of my best physical features—an opinion shared by my husband. Losing a breast damaged my self-image to a certain extent, especially after I discovered that the implant was a poor substitute. I have only gradually come to see that what mother said is really true—the people who count love my body because they love my soul, no matter how misshapen that body may appear to me.

Of course, I could remedy the lopsidedness by having the left breast removed. The doctor feels this would be appropriate, since it received just as much radiation as the right breast and could develop cancer as well, even though he biopsied it at the time of the implant and it looked normal. There is a certain amount of risk involved in keeping it, although he assures me that changes would be easy to catch. Because of this, I have resisted another mastectomy for several reasons, such as the loss of sensation and the unwillingness to undergo more surgery and further mutilation. Although I may decide later that I am tired of living lopsided, right now it seems to be important to me to stubbornly require the rest of the world to accept my body on my terms.

Or it may be to get myself to accept it. Both rounds of cancer have created within me very ambivalent feelings about my body. I've never really forgiven it for developing Hodgkin's disease at such an inopportune time. However, after producing two children, we seemed to be developing a better alliance. At the time the breast cancer was discovered, my body was in the best shape of my life. I had been working out three times a week for a couple of years, was eating very carefully, and now weighed less than when I got married. So I felt a double sense of betrayal when it developed cancer again. I didn't react very sanely—I quit exercising, started eating comfort foods (chocolate, French fries, wine), and, of course, eventually gained twenty pounds. Only recently have I started working out again, partly as a result of writing this chapter. When I first started lifting weights, I had visions of the implant popping out and flying across the room, but it seems to be firmly in place. It's interesting to discover that, although the surgery was on the right side, it's the muscles on the left side of my upper body that need the most work.

Even when working out, I am rarely conscious of being lopsided. When I see myself in a mirror, I think, "Oh, yeah, that's right, one side's larger." I have to buy clothes very carefully and have put away some of my clingiest sweaters. But mostly my mind is on other things. Like life.

. . . .

Walking the line

Developing cancer is like becoming a parent for the first time—you know it's irreversible, but you don't know how it will affect your life. It takes time to come to terms with the change and to discover where the consequences will show up. For example, I found out last year that I am virtually uninsurable. Fortunately, my husband's health insurance covers me fully and has been excellent about doing so. But life insurance is prohibitively expensive and disability insurance is unavailable for at least five more years.

Another unknown is the effect this has on our children. The younger daughter, now nine, asks me, "Mommy, why did they cut off your breast?" I try to explain that it had a disease and that we had to take it off before it spread to the rest of my body. And I wonder, "Will she worry now that if she breaks an arm, we're going to cut it off?" I worry more about the older daughter, because she has much more sense of what the disease could mean. I don't think she broods about it, but for her, as for us, it's always there.

The major consequences, however, are emotional. I have discovered several "fine lines" that have to be walked very carefully in order to live a normal life. First, there is a fine line between disregarding messages from your body and falling into rampant hypochondria. You have to learn to pay attention to your physical condition without worrying that every little pain could be the start of something big. I've found that anxiety attacks usually happen in the dead of night. I wake up for some reason and lie there, full of dread, feeling every ache, wondering if I'll see my kids grow up. After the ritual half hour or so of panic and self-pity, I remind myself that I have survived some pretty tough blows already and that I will survive a recurrence emotionally and probably physically as well. Then I relax my body, repeat the Twenty-third Psalm, and remember the garlic presses.

There is another compromise between blatant self-indulgence and refusal to modify your life in any way. You have to treat yourself with the same consideration you would give a loved one in the same situation. On the one hand, say no when you want to. Give yourself special treats. Relax. Don't be too hard on yourself when you are not perfect. But at the same time, realize that having cancer is not an excuse for grabbing everything you can get now. Normal life does require discipline and some delay of gratification.

Another balancing act is between self-pity (why did this happen to me? I don't deserve this) and guilt (I must have done something wrong; it's all my fault). You have to separate taking responsibility for your reactions to the disease, which you can control, and feeling guilty for having the disease, which you are not responsible for. One of the wisest things my first doctor said was, "Don't waste any time wondering why it happened or what caused it. We don't know, and you need your strength for other things."

Another, more insidious, problem is the role the disease comes to have in your life. You can do a macho act, pretending it was no big deal, no harder to cope with than the common cold. But then you rob yourself of the credit of facing and surviving a very difficult physical and spiritual ordeal. On the other hand, it is very easy to begin to feel "special" because you have survived and to think that other people should regard you as special too. Of course, it is an intense experience that shaped the person you have become, and the people who care for you need to know about it and will value your achievement (the people who don't care about you may not be as sympathetic). The danger here is that you can come to regard the encounter with cancer as the most important event in your life and be unable to let go of it emotionally. It can become the way you define yourself as a person, which negates the other aspects of your being, the other strengths and accomplishments and joys.

The final consequence I want to mention is that growing old takes on a new meaning. Each birthday becomes a cause for celebration rather than a trauma. When I turned forty, we gave a huge party to celebrate the ten years that had passed since the Hodgkin's disease. We invited all the many friends who had shared our lives during that ten-year period. It was a lovely evening. I'm already looking forward to my fiftieth birthday—it's going to be one hell of a party.

Second Pair $1

David Mickelsen (Vicki's husband)

I was a bystander. The knife didn't slice my skin, and I lost no flesh. I didn't face mortality directly. However, these matters have a way of involving the "spectators." To turn the term around, I did stand by—not as a helpless spectator, but as a support; I tried to stand by my wife during her breast-cancer experience.

It is from this perspective, then, that I can discuss two topics: how I responded during my wife's diagnosis and treatment, and how surgery has affected our sexual relationship. What follows is a description rather than a prescription.

First, you should know that I'm an optimist (which is a good deal easier when you're not the one with the disease). I don't dwell on the past; thus, I tend to put unpleasant situations rapidly behind me. In this case, however, optimism was not unreasonable. Vicki had already coped successfully with Hodgkin's disease fourteen years earlier. To contract cancer a second time might be depressing, and, of course, it was, but it also equipped us with a kind of optimism: we knew you could get cancer and survive (never mind that the radiation treatment for the first cancer probably caused the second).

In other ways, too, this second occurrence was easier, since it had an even better cure rate than Hodgkin's (Vicki had at least managed to contract only the most treatable of cancers), and this time we had none of the wrenching complications of pregnancy. Even the postoperative treatment was easier, since neither radiation nor chemotherapy was prescribed. Thus, aside from the short-term effects of the mastectomy, nothing interrupted the workings of optimism—an optimism that was reinforced, I might add, by full confidence in the doctor in charge of her care.

Perhaps it is easy for survivors, for those whose stories have happy endings, to recall the good parts and neglect the bad. Be that as it may, I still think that fear and depression figured importantly in my attitudes at the time.

Having few fears about the success of the treatment, I occupied myself with "standing by"—with making that treatment as manageable and bearable as possible. I wanted to be understanding of the pains without making them the center of our existence. I tried to be matter-of-fact about them, almost businesslike, because I was convinced they were just a temporary, albeit inconvenient, part of our lives. My policy was to keep a low profile while staying "available." I tried to be supportive in terms of demands and responsibilities, but in a light, rather than lugubrious, manner. I sent her into biopsy surgery with dotted lines and "Cut Here" inked on her chest. For the mastectomy itself, I gave her a sign, salvaged from a shoe ad, which read "Second Pair $1." Lest you think I'm completely without scruple, please note that I recently resisted commenting on the appropriateness of Vicki attending a conference in Silicon Valley.

We were fortunate in having a surgeon with buoyant, even boyish, good spirits. Even if he failed to see the humor in his blithely nonchalant use of such words as "oncophobic" and "nulliparity," he tolerated our bemusement and was indulgent when we laughed at his deadpan statement, while speaking of mammography, that Vicki has a "followable breast." He even endured a laudatory limerick:

Incisive Comments

> When Hogle arrives to repair
>   a cancerous breast or a pair,
>   well-reasoned decisions
>   precede all incisions—
> you know how what when why and where.

Aside from his obvious professional skill, he remained unfailingly upbeat without sacrificing candor. His infectious (if you will) good nature reinforced my own inclination to be optimistic, which might have been more difficult with a surgeon less informative and supportive. The following poem, provoked by the reconstructive process, is supposed to convey that sense of concord, despite its Lizzy Borden rhythm.

The Fall and Rise of a Woman's Empire
or
Keeping Abreast

> Hughie Hogle took a knife,
> wielded it upon my wife,

pared her pair, reduced the fat
from hill to plain in nothing flat.

Now he's back, with manic grin,
ready to inflate, not trim.
Can a maimed and furrowed chest
rise again at his behest?

In a reconstructed future
surely all will laud his suture.
Hughie Hogle, he's the best—
deftest scalpel in the West.

The mastectomy itself took place during Christmas vacation, not an obviously opportune moment, but one which actually offered a multitude of distractions. In addition to being a period free of work pressures, family and friends were easily available. I'm not sure they always shared my conviction that while this was serious, it wasn't threatening, but they too tended to be attentive without directly addressing the issue of disease. They too were part of the necessary corps of those standing by.

During the postoperative period, my involvement has diminished, and I have become more truly a bystander. As an inner-directed person, Vicki has drawn for support on a range of books rather than on personal interaction. I have been more sympathetic to some of these than to others, though I have tried, perhaps not always successfully, to preserve a strict neutrality. For me, the important issue has been the practical utility of the books, rather than their abstract validity. Have they helped her cope or not?

I have maintained a similar neutrality concerning further prophylactic and cosmetic surgery. Although only one breast was affected, Dr. Hogle recommended a double mastectomy as a precaution, but Vicki has preferred not to pursue that option. That decision agrees perfectly with my optimistic outlook, but I follow her lead, let her make the choices. Likewise, she has chosen not to have further reconstructive surgery after the initial implant, even though her appearance is fairly obviously asymmetrical. Again, I fully support the decision she's most comfortable with—after all, she's the one who has to live with the consequences (she found a prosthesis to be too cumbersome and, understandably, doesn't relish further surgery).

This leads to the second and briefer of my topics: What does a guy raised in *Playboy* America do when his wife loses a breast? For me, the answer was easy. The question always rapidly transmuted to, "What does a guy do if he loses his wife?" The choice was that simple—the breast or the wife. Those pounds of flesh were a small price to pay. I helped remove the bandages for the first time after the mastectomy, and I wasn't at all shocked or dismayed. In context, it didn't matter. Now, this might seem to be a rather simpleminded approach, and perhaps that's a source of my optimism. I'm not inclined to introspection, as this chapter probably suggests. In any case, for me, the choices were uncomplicated.

Seduction, it is often said, is more mental than physical, and I can vouch for that. Were I to wax philosophical, I'd argue that American attitudes toward women fixate on the surface (surely the aerobics fad has more to do with that than with health), and, of course, breasts have been a prominent locus of attention. Ironically, this was especially true for Vicki; "generously endowed," a prim cliche, was not inflated rhetoric in her case. Yet even though that attraction has been, well, reapportioned, lovemaking has certainly not become less enjoyable for me. In part, the disease itself contributes to the trivialization of the surface—recovery becomes so important that details of contour and volume are reduced (literally, if I may say) to minor status. Whatever the reason, in terms of the attraction of one person to another, in this particular case, I find that altered topography does not result in altered ardor.

Having said what I have to say, I wonder if it really conveys all that needs to be conveyed. Words fail; cases vary. Perhaps this more serious poem, while referring to a specific moment now many years ago, will provide as good a conclusion as any:

Partition

The night before
they took your breast,
we parted with that part
by making love.
You knew we would,
and so did I,
but no words passed.
Instead we lay
before the fire
and put that ache
into each other's arms
instead of words.

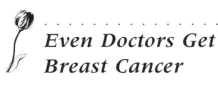

Even Doctors Get Breast Cancer

K. Mack, M.D.

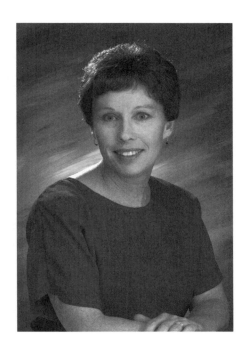

Dr. K. Mack, a physician specializing in internal medicine, writes under a pseudonym to protect her privacy. Dr. Mack and her husband are devoted to their work and live a quiet life, reading and making plans for their adventurous trips. Dr. Mack particularly emphasizes educating her patients about their bodies and has gained sensitivity to them because of her own experiences. In particular, she is aware of the emotional and physical cost of "routine" tests and the anxiety of waiting for results. She included her medical biography here because "in my daily contact with patients I try to keep in mind that every line in their chart may represent chapters of their lives."

Medical Bio

In September 1985, at age thirty-two, Dr. Mack noticed a lump in the lower outer portion of her left breast. She had previously been diagnosed and treated for cancer of the thyroid gland. A needle aspiration after the discovery of the mass showed no evidence of breast cancer. Shortly after Thanksgiving, because of the persistence of the mass, a biopsy was done that showed a medullary cancer of the breast. She elected to have breast conservation and went back to surgery, where the axillary lymph nodes were removed. One of them was positive for metastatic breast cancer. She then completed a course of radiation therapy and a course of chemotherapy.

Approximately one year later, she noticed another lump in her previously treated left breast. By January 1987, the lump had enlarged somewhat, and small skin eruptions were beginning to appear on the breast. A biopsy of one of these skin lesions showed metastatic breast cancer. A biopsy of the mass also showed it to be a recurrent breast cancer. Dr. Mack was returned to surgery, where she underwent a left mastectomy and wide local excision of all of the skin lesions. She had another course of radiation therapy with hyperthermia and was started on Tamoxifen.

She remained well until March 1988, when she discovered a 1.5-centimeter lump in her right armpit. A biopsy identified metastatic breast cancer. After extensive consultation, the decision was made to carry out a right modified radical mastectomy, which was accomplished in April 1988. On pathologic examination of the right breast and axillary contents, no breast cancer could be identified, either in the breast or in the remaining axillary nodes. She has had no further signs of breast cancer recurrence. She has chosen not to have reconstruction done.

I asked my husband, "What is this bump on the back of my arm?" I couldn't quite see it, and I held my arm out for him to look at it. To my surprise, he reached beyond my arm and touched my breast (which would have normally started another sort of activity!) and asked me what I thought this other little lump was. At first, I didn't feel what he was referring to, but then it came into tactile "focus" under my fingertips. It felt about the size of a grapefruit seed and seemed almost gritty as I moved it over my rib, which was the only way I could really feel it. As a physician, I tried to analyze the situation. I did not know of any family history of this type of cancer, so my only risk factor was that I had not had children. This information should have been reassuring, but something deep inside told me that this was going to be big trouble. I had never noticed this little voice before, but I was going to find that it would be amazingly accurate when it spoke.

During that sleepless night, I could not get the thought of cancer out of my mind. This was too reminiscent of an experience I had had about four years earlier. At that time, I was studying for my medical boards and found a lump in my neck. It turned out to be cancer. Well, I was now within ten days of another board exam!

The next morning, I maintained my composure through rounds at the hospital; almost anything is possible behind that professional smile. As soon as I hit the office and shut the door, I called a surgical colleague for advice. I knew I had a healthy imagination. I also knew what needed to be done medically, but someone else would have to orchestrate it. I was unable to convince myself that the lump I had felt was real.

I went over to the surgeon's office, and we checked it out before my office duties started. I squeezed in a mammogram and an ultrasound between patients and meetings during the day. The mammogram was negative but the ultrasound showed the lump to be solid—even though I was wishing with all my might that it would be cystic. A few days later, the surgeon aspirated the nodule with a needle. That was okay until the novocaine wore off and I was still seeing patients.

The needle aspirate was negative! I sat for the exam with a clear head a few days later.

The lump persisted, and an open biopsy was planned for Friday, two days past my birthday. I had taken off work on my birthday and gone hiking and had one of the most glorious days in the mountains I'd ever had. I did not even think of the biopsy that day.

After the biopsy on Friday morning, I was lying in the recovery room trying to get my senses together enough to say something funny to the nurses when my surgeon walked in. The look on his face was somewhere between shock and horror. It was breast cancer. The word echoed for a long time in my sedated head. I felt like I was trying to fight off an invisible enemy with the coordination one has in a dream. As I recovered from the anesthesia, everyone was very nice, but no one came in to tell me that the original diagnosis was a mistake and that the official report was negative for malignancy.

I called my family, but my husband had to tell them, because I couldn't say the word *cancer* without crying.

I spent hours with my surgeons and my oncologist. They patiently went over every option with me and my husband. They encouraged me to read or call anyone I knew to help me decide the course of therapy. I called some physicians who I knew and trusted, and talked to them about the pros and cons of the treatments my physicians and I were considering. I was looking for that little piece of data that would give me a better chance of being cured. I also talked to two women with breast cancer who had made two different choices about their treatment. After all the medical and personal discussions and a lot of thinking, the two choices remained equal. Should it be the lumpectomy and radiation or the mastectomy?

I chose the lumpectomy with axillary dissection and radiation. It seemed to be less invasive to my body. Surgery was performed, and an unexpected positive node was found in the axillary dissection. The treatment plan was modified to include chemotherapy. This plan sounded like a good, aggressive approach, and I was in the mood to get this taken care of and behind me. The tumor was small, and there was only one node microscopically involved. Statistically, it was not so bad.

. . . .

Chemotherapy, radiation therapy, river therapy

Chemotherapy started first. I took some blue-and-white pills daily and two yellow injections in the vein weekly. I felt like I had a low-grade flu that I could not shake. My hair thinned, but it wasn't noticeable to anyone but close friends.

Radiation therapy started within a few days of chemotherapy. It soon became routine. Grab a locker key (I was always late), wrap the gown around me twice, make sure it was tied securely, and sit down and try to look like a visitor. Between visits, I wore silk long underwear to protect my skin from my clothes and protect my clothes from the black indelible marker lines on my chest.

The fatiguing effects of radiation decreased a few weeks after the treatments. Shortly after that, I began to experience an "electrical" feeling in my feet and legs, especially if I bent my neck forward. I was sure that this was a sign of spinal cord metastatic cancer. When I finally got the courage to call the doctor with this "devastating" news, it did not evoke the serious response I had thought it would. He laughed! And then he explained that I had beautifully described a rare syndrome called LeHermettes Syndrome and that it would go away. And it did, eventually.

More good news: I passed the medical boards!

Even when the radiation was over, the chemotherapy continued to give me a low-grade-flu feeling, but my husband and I decided to go ahead with the outdoor adventures that we had always enjoyed. The first one that I distinctly remember was a river trip in Oregon. We launched in a drizzle, which became a downpour as the afternoon went on. I was just happy to be back out on a river and away from doctors' offices. There is nothing like paddling to make you aware of the importance of a full range of motion in the shoulder. The paddling improved the strength in my arms almost as much as pulling the required layers of clothing and gear off and on as needed to empty my bladder. One of my chemotherapy drugs required that I stay very well hydrated, and I didn't want to have any problems on the trip. Well, the weather improved, and my stream-side excursions were less chilling. The trip was a real confidence builder for me. The people, scenery, and activity were outstanding for someone who had been spending too much time in clinics and hospitals of late.

A few weeks later, I noticed that I was more fatigued than usual and it took me longer to get ready for work, but I thought that it was all in my head. When it got to the point that I was too tired to even talk to myself in full sentences, I knew that there was definitely something wrong. My oncologist was out of town, so I called my radiation oncologist to see if the problem was possibly related to the radiation. I knew that radiation could sometimes cause inflammation in the lungs. Going to the radiation center, I felt like I was moving in slow motion. After the tests were taken, I was told that I had hypoxemia (low on oxygen in the bloodstream) and I needed to be in the hospital. I was treated with steroids and improved quickly over the next few days.

All the sympathy and attention were nice, but I wanted this whole thing to be over. I'm the type of person who likes to get things done and put them in neat little piles. It didn't seem so bad: a few surgeries, radiation, chemotherapy, and a couple of unusual complications. Why then was it so hard to deal with? Why couldn't I sleep? Why did I cry so easily? Why couldn't life get back to the way it had been before cancer? I had been given some of those self-help books and tapes, but there were so many conflicting ideas— meditation, interpersonal communication, trust, assertiveness, fantasy, facts. I took this to mean that no one knew how to help us get better. Drawing pictures didn't seem strong enough, but joining a group was too much for me. I needed to talk about it but keep my privacy. I was worried about what would happen to me professionally. Therefore, I confided in some close friends and family. Everyone stayed so positive; they brought me more books and video tapes, sent me to conferences, and kept me in their plans. They put up with my slow skiing, slow hiking, and some tears. These things helped, but it was still going to take time.

I was frustrated. After the radiation and with the ongoing chemotherapy, I couldn't keep up my previous work and activity schedule. This was an entirely new concept to me. I needed to make some choices. I decided again to make sure that I took enough time for myself, just as I had vowed not to work too hard and take time for myself after my mother's death (at the same time as my previous cancer). In reading the self-help books, I now realized that I needed to choose the techniques that were right for me. I also had to be fair to the patients and the other doctors who depended on me. There was (is) no easy answer, and I'm still working on this conflict.

One choice that I had made was to try to run the Colorado River through the Grand Canyon, if it was possible with my current medical situation. One day during chemotherapy infusions, I mentioned this proposed adventure—two-and-a-half weeks in the Grand Canyon by kayak—to my oncologist. I had been looking forward to this trip for seven years. Late in spring, it was obvious that I would still be on chemotherapy when we were to leave. My oncologist, an outdoor enthusiast himself, thought it would be a good (no, great) trip for me to do. When the launch date came, I was in good health—so we set off down the canyon. It started off easily, mainly in calm water. Then came the rapids, loud, wet, exhilarating, and scary. I felt somewhat invincible in view of what I had just survived, but, nonetheless, I was careful. So what if I walked around some of the rapids and napped on a raft on an afternoon or two? Conversations no longer revolved around statistics, chemo, X-rays, or blood tests; the main topics were the rapids, campsites, and the next meal.

The chemotherapy finally ended. I kind of missed it, in the way that you miss a very hard teacher and are glad for the lessons you've learned.

. . . .
First the left breast . . .

Autumn came and we hiked in the glorious colors. Ski racks were appearing on cars, signaling the start of winter and the frozen-winter adventures. It had been a year since it had all started. As I toasted to my health on the anniversary of my diagnosis, there was a nagging doubt in my mind about my health. I had discovered some bumps in the radiation area on my chest. My worst suspicions were confirmed when they quickly multiplied in several areas and on biopsy were found to contain breast-cancer cells.

A mastectomy was scheduled. The blood tests and nuclear scans were negative, showing no evidence of cancer elsewhere. The night before surgery we made love, because I knew that this was the last time I'd make love with two breasts.

I woke up from surgery feeling like I was wrapped too tight. The surgeons had skillfully removed all the skin lesions with the breast and wrapped the wound up tight. The hospital tumor board recommended either repeat "surface" radiation and Tamoxifen or a new course of chemotherapy. I felt that the Tamoxifen therapy was nonaggressive, but when I found out that estrogen receptors were positive and that the data on survival were about the same for both treatments, I went for the Tamoxifen.

Radiation this time consisted of lying under the machine as before but with the addition of a new machine. This machine was described as being like a microwave that would augment the effect of the radiation by warming the radiation site. I sort of felt like a leftover being put in to reheat.

Radiation wasn't the only thing warming me; the Tamoxifen had started causing hot flashes. I found these to be very useful in the winter but a bother in the summer.

Winter flashed by (pun intended) with the usual work and ski trips. A minor case of the dreaded shingles (herpes zoster) tried to slow me down, but I had quite a few ski passes to use up.

The snow began to melt, and soon we were ready for summer adventures. For variety, we went on a bicycle tour in Europe with some relatives of mine. We also had another opportunity to run the Colorado River in the Grand Canyon in late summer. I did not feel as invincible this time, nor was I as tired.

At the same time, I was also working a lot.

In that season when you put away the toys of summer and get the winter toys waxed and sharpened, I found some lumps above my left collarbone. I'd had a recent insect bite on that arm, and my oncologist and I decided to watch the lumps. Then came some little, wart-like growths in the radiation field. Deja vu? The biopsy report was short: warts, common warts. My first negative biopsy!

Spring and summer were quite uneventful medically but full of the things of summer: hiking, boating, beautiful sunsets. My family and friends no longer dreaded hearing from me as there was occasional good news.

In the fall, after an especially rigorous month at work, I started having abdominal pains. After an extensive evaluation, including blood tests, CT scans, and a needle aspirate of my abdominal fluid, the problem was narrowed down to my ovaries. I was sent to a gynecologic oncologist for presumed breast-cancer recurrence around the ovaries. The little voice inside me told me that this was not cancer. I then hypothesized that the Tamoxifen had caused the ovarian swellings. A complete hysterectomy was scheduled. In a few days, surgery confirmed my diagnosis. The case was written up for the medical journals as the first of its kind.

. . . .

And then the right breast . . .

The next excitement came in the shower. Innocently soaping up one day, I found a lump in my right armpit. (Everything had been on the left side so far.) I resolved not to get overexcited, as I felt I'd had my fair share of this disease and was a little cocky in view of my previously negative biopsy and surgery. I did bring it to the oncologist's attention, and a biopsy was scheduled.

It was positive. My inner voice was wrong on this one—or did I just not want to believe it? The only logical course as far as I was concerned was a mastectomy.

I made love that night for the last time with a breast.

This was a more traditional surgery in terms of the scar. About ten days later, I rode in a bikeathon. It seemed that my body had taken quite seriously a comment that I had made to a friend many years ago. We had been lamenting our less-than-perfect figures, and I said that I knew I would never have a classic Barbie-doll body but would be happy with a good functional body. I didn't mean that I would have *minded* a Barbie-doll body that functioned well.

Reconstructive breast surgery was offered, but in my case, with two different surgeries and high-dose radiation therapies, it would have been an involved process. I just couldn't face more surgeries. I wear traditional silicon breast prostheses for in-town activities and cheaper, more durable, and easily replaceable prostheses for camping and adventures.

The trips and the diversions were fine, but what did it all mean? The tests, chemotherapy, radiation, surgeries, recoveries, then recurrences kept me always reevaluating my life and priorities. I was taking the time to appreciate things that I valued and trying to do all the right things, but the cancer kept recurring. Medical science, which I was heavily invested in personally, did not seem able to check this cancer. The Tamoxifen had been discontinued because the right breast axillary lesion was reportedly a sign of its ineffectiveness. It was all up to me now, and I realized that it had been all along. Even though my brain was sometimes caught up in a muddle of statistics and jargon, my body had consistently chosen to live and heal.

Seven months later, we headed out on a day hike, which ended up as an unexpected overnight hike. We bivouacked and had a long second day with little food or water. I used techniques that I had used during therapy: focusing attention on what I was doing (while ignoring the cliff below me) and acknowledging my fear but not letting it overcome my ability to function. The physical reserve that I had taken for granted before cancer and that was conspicuously absent during treatment was back. I had a personal welcome-home party to celebrate its return.

There have been some more trips and a few scares of cancer recurrences since, but I am still here. I do not consider myself exceptional. I did what I needed to do to survive. I think that my doctors, family, friends, and especially my husband are exceptional. Many thanks to them all, and to my husband for the hours of back rubs.

Go for it . . .

An Alternative Form of Early Detection

Tim Rule (Dr. K. Mack's husband)

It was quite accidental and natural that I should have found the lump in my wife's breast. We both enjoyed holding and touching each other as part of lovemaking. Consequently, I spent more time touching her breasts than the most rigorous self-examination schedule would require. I expect that this would apply to many couples. While we were making love, I naturally was not checking for anything unusual. And because of the passion of the moment, I did not mention it at the time. In fact, I did not remember the lump until some time later when my wife asked me about some bump she had noticed on her skin. She was very upset by my revelation that there was a lump in her breast. I was not as concerned at the time. The difference in our reactions is that she immediately thought of the worst that it could be, while I thought it most likely was not cancer, and, if it were, it could be cured. Also, it was late in the evening, and we could not do anything immediately.

I share this experience in the hope that it might encourage another man who has noticed a lump in his wife or partner to tell her and encourage her to have it checked immediately by a doctor. I have tried to analyze why I mentioned the lump instead of passing it off as unimportant, but I cannot think of anything specific that influenced me. I had been exposed to small doses of cancer education for a long time; I can recall that there are seven signs of cancer, but I cannot name all of them. I know that early detection and treatment are the key to cure. I also know that there is a technique of breast self-examination for women, but I do not know the details. If I happened to be practicing any of the right techniques when I discovered my wife's tumor, it was purely coincidental. Realizing this made me wonder if there would be a benefit to teaching husbands how to check for lumps in their wives' breasts. It might help detect some cases of cancer at an earlier state.

After my wife calmed down from the initial thought that the lump in her breast might be cancer, she had it checked. The initial tests, mammography, and needle biopsy were negative. These were reassuring results, but to be completely certain, she scheduled a biopsy to remove the lump and have a complete pathology report.

The biopsy went smoothly, but the initial pathology report was delayed. The surgeon felt the lump was benign based on the appearance, so he closed the incision before the pathology report was complete to prevent my wife from being under anesthesia longer than necessary. He was noticeably shocked when he told me the results were positive and that he had probably offended the pathologist by questioning the report. It is hard to describe how I felt at this point. I tried to concentrate on the fact that the cancer had been detected early and could be cured.

After we found out that the lump was malignant, we had a brief time to choose a course of treatment. We felt it desirable to take enough time to evaluate all the options and feel comfortable with the decision. However, it is hard to know what is enough time and what is too much. Medically, neither option was significantly better than the other. Both had undesirable side effects, and neither gave us the certainty we wanted: the guarantee of a permanent cure. The only thing we knew was that either option was better than doing nothing.

We selected the least disfiguring option of lumpectomy and nodectomy followed by radiation and chemotherapy. A few months after completing chemotherapy, my wife noticed some bumps on the skin of her breast. It turned out that they were cancerous. The only option at this point was a mastectomy of the left breast and more radiation. About a year later, she found a lump in her right armpit. This time the treatment was mastectomy and nodectomy on the right side, followed by chemotherapy. The final episode was a side effect of the latest chemotherapy: an infarcted ovary, which was treated by the removal of her ovaries and a hysterectomy.

The most devastating time for me was after my wife found the lump in her right armpit. The doctors disagreed about the significance of that event; the surgeon said that it was still a local disease and probably could be cured by surgery, while the oncologist felt that it meant the disease had spread. When he said that the reason for treatment at that point was to keep the best quality of life possible, I interpreted his words to mean, "Be prepared for the worst." I found it difficult to maintain an optimistic outlook. I tried to remember the surgeon's advice and hoped for the best. We are now well beyond the time frame that the oncologist had projected at the time, and she has had no more signs of cancer. This taught me to keep a doctor's prognosis in perspective. Doctors do not claim to know how a particular case will progress. All a medical prognosis can do is give statistics about what has happened to groups of people in similar situations.

The treatment was difficult. Surgeries, radiation, and chemotherapy took their toll. To combat these effects, I encouraged my wife to work at a reduced level, and I planned activities to give her goals after the treatment. We had been active in outdoor sports before the cancer, so I planned kayak trips, cross-country ski trips, a bicycle trip, and backpacking. We also scheduled more leisurely visits to her family scattered around Wisconsin, Tennessee, Germany, and Mexico. Some of the trips took place very soon after the treatments, and she needed to take it easier than she had before the treatments. Her lack of energy discouraged her at times, but she did show that she could still do the same things as before.

Now, two years later, the only reminders of cancer are the regular checkups and the uncertainty of the ultimate effect of the treatment.

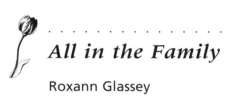

All in the Family

Roxann Glassey

Roxann is the proud mother of four boys and part of a large and supportive extended family. She has been closely involved in community activities, most recently as PTA president of a local elementary school. Roxann works part-time as a skin-care consultant and devotes herself to her children and to her religion.

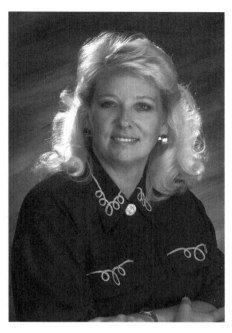

Her favorite activity is attending her teenagers' basketball and football games. She and her husband, John, particularly enjoy family boating trips. Religion is fundamental to Roxann. She reads religious novels and plays in church-sponsored sports leagues. Recently, she and two friends founded a T-shirt company called "MoraliTees," which prints and sells T-shirts with positive messages.

Medical Bio

Roxann has a strong family history of breast cancer, including the fact that her mother experienced the disease at age forty-one. She had been participating in a high-risk program and was having a routine mammogram in October 1989 when microcalcifications were discovered in the left breast. A breast biopsy was accomplished, and the pathology showed intraductal and microinvasive cancer of the left breast. She underwent a left modified radical mastectomy and also chose to have a right simple mastectomy. Both were

accomplished with immediate bilateral subpectoral prosthetic breast reconstructions.

The cancer in her left breast proved to be a 2.5-centimeter tumor.
None of the twenty-one lymph nodes removed showed signs of metastatic
cancer. She is now well with no signs of recurrent breast cancer and has experienced no problems subsequent to her bilateral breast reconstructions.

I guess I knew deep down inside that it would happen to me, but is
anyone prepared to hear the word *cancer* in reference to herself? My mother
had a mastectomy fifteen years ago. At that time I was twenty-one years old
and could not imagine myself in that scenario. That was a time when I thought
that I was totally invincible and the words, "that will never happen to me,"
came into my conversation frequently. As I got older, and some things did
happen to me, I became aware of my mortality.

This was brought home to me eleven years after my mother's diagnosis when my thirty-two-year-old cousin was not only diagnosed with breast
cancer but died six months later. How could this happen? She was so young!
She left three beautiful children and a grieving husband. Mom had five sisters
and each of them had several daughters. It scared all of us. We all promised to
get the dreaded mammogram. It's tough, you know, to go that first time. All
our lives we are taught modesty, and here we had to stand in front of a
stranger bare-chested. At least the technician was female, it didn't hurt, and
it wasn't nearly as embarrassing as a pelvic exam! So we all braved it and
found out it wasn't so bad. All of us, that is, except one aunt.

She knew she had a lump in her breast, and she was scared to go for
fear of what they might find. The sisters all checked with each other to make
sure each one had the mammogram. It was easier for my aunt to say she
had gone than to face the results. Finally she admitted to one sister that she
was scared, and we basically forced her to see a doctor.

It was cancer, and it had progressed quite far. No wonder she was
scared. If only she had been able to face it earlier, things wouldn't be so tough
now. She did have a mastectomy and now endures radiation and chemotherapy treatments. The cancer is in remission, but she lives each day with a prayer
in her heart that the cancer has not spread to other parts of her body.

When a local university called my family in September 1989 and asked
us to be part of a clinical-research study on breast cancer in relation to
mother/daughter heredity, we quickly accepted. Mom, my sister, and I had a
nice time together that day. We enjoyed seeing each other, a rare event since
my sister had moved away.

However, three days later the lab called me and said there was something wrong with my mammogram. Would I please come back for a follow-up check? I was sure there was some mistake because I had been having no trouble; I never even told Mom about it because I knew she would worry. But after they had me repeat the mammogram three times, I finally began to get nervous. They did find something, even though there was no detectable lump. The doctor wanted a biopsy of the area to find out what it was.

After the biopsy, I was so worried that I called repeatedly for three days trying to find out results. Finally, the doctor called and said he had wanted to wait to speak to me until our appointment in two days; he didn't want to tell me the news on the phone. But since I had been so persistent, he decided to return my call. As he told me that I did have breast cancer, I felt I couldn't hold myself up. I don't know how I did it, but I remained very calm on the phone and listened to all he had to say. Then I called my husband, John, at work. That's when I fell apart. I was sobbing so hard he could hardly understand me. But he knew.

At that moment, I desperately needed someone to hold me and let me cry. John was at least twenty minutes away, and I didn't want to scare my boys. As I hung up the phone, my younger brother, who had been worried about me, walked in the front door. He didn't say anything. He just held me and let me cry until John got home.

The next few weeks were filled with fear and decisions. At the appointment with the doctor, he explained that the biopsy sample had cancer cells scattered throughout, and we needed to make a decision as to what we should do. He said that there were several options. There could not be a lumpectomy because there was no lump. The cancer had invaded the tissue and was scattered throughout the breast. He told me that I could have the entire breast radiated and that there was a chance that all of the cancer would be killed. Another option was a mastectomy with nodectomy. Reconstructive surgery at the same time as the mastectomy was also a possibility. This would require the plastic surgeon to coordinate with the general surgeon during the surgery.

John and I were very confused and scared. I knew that I did not feel comfortable with the idea of radiation therapy. I was afraid that the cancer might not be killed by the radiation, and I couldn't live with the fear. We decided that we would like a second opinion. A neighbor told me about a very good doctor who would be willing to look at the X-rays and give his opinion of the situation. I called the first doctor, and he was very cooperative in getting all X-rays, reports, and biopsy slides released to the new doctor.

The second doctor agreed with the first diagnosis. He gave me the same options as the first doctor, but because he was a breast-care specialist, he was qualified to do both the mastectomy and the reconstructive surgery. After two hours of discussion, he told us to talk about it for a few days and then call him and tell him the decision we had made.

I don't need to tell you that this subject was the only thing we could think or talk about for the next three days. We talked to others who had gone through breast cancer, including my mother. We read booklets from the American Cancer Society. We also prayed a lot and listened to our feelings. Finally, it was time to give the doctor our decision. After all the thinking, talking, reading, and praying, the decision I made was to have not just a mastectomy but a double mastectomy. I wanted to be rid of the cancer, and I didn't want to live with the fear that it would recur in my right breast. John felt that whatever would make me feel comfortable would be the best thing for us. I was afraid that the doctor would not agree with this drastic measure. When I first presented him with my decision, he did say that he felt it was a bit of "overkill," but given my family history, he said that we could go for it.

I wanted to get everything done RIGHT NOW. Now that I knew that the cancer was there and what I wanted to do about it, I wanted it out of my body so that it could not have a chance to grow any more. Life definitely takes on a different perspective when you are faced with cancer surgery. Some of the things that were so important before seem ridiculous, and it is hard to believe that you were even worried about such trivial things.

The doctor told me not to panic. He told me that the cancer had probably been growing for a couple of years and wouldn't even be to the lump stage for another two years. Even though cancer is a fast-growing disease, he convinced me that, at this stage, a few days or even weeks would not make a life-threatening difference.

A few obstacles did get in the way before surgery. My doctor wanted a pint of my own blood to be available in case of emergency. I had a cold sore, which I get when I am nervous, and they could not take my blood until it was healed. I was so afraid to wait that I convinced the doctor to take a pint of my father's blood. Even though I knew that the time was not that critical, each extra day of waiting was agony to me. I was not afraid of the surgery. I was not even worried about losing my breasts. I just couldn't bear the thought of the cancer growing inside of me.

On November 8, 1989, I entered the hospital for my surgery. The doctor had told me that the surgery would take about six or seven hours. He would remove the breast tissue in both breasts, the lymph nodes from under each arm, and then implant a silicone-gel bag in each side that would later be filled with saline. I had chosen to have implants done at the same time, because I felt that it would be easier for me to accept the scars if my chest were at least still round and soft.

The surgery took about six-and-a-half hours, and everything went beautifully. The breast tissue was removed from both breasts, along with twenty-one lymph nodes from the left side and four from the right side. The doctor said that the cancer had spread throughout the left breast and that the right one had precancerous cells. This made me feel even better about my decision to have both breasts removed.

I had the surgery on Wednesday. By Friday I was up and around and ready to go home by 9:30 A.M. When the surgical nurse came in to release me, she told me to keep the area tightly wrapped, not to get it wet, and to empty the drains that were on either side. She then informed me that all lymph nodes had come back negative. The relief is impossible to convey in words. It was the most exciting news I had had in five weeks. My mother was so relieved, she actually broke down and sobbed. In my case, the negative reports meant that there would be no radiation or chemotherapy.

My mother admitted to me how terrified she had been for me. She had been very supportive and concerned, but she was careful not to let me see the fear she felt. It took most of her courage to keep this from me so that I wouldn't be so frightened while I was going through it. My experience was bringing back many terrifying feelings she had felt fifteen years ago, but she didn't want my fear to be multiplied by hers. Several times she told me that if she could have gone through it for me, she would have. She said watching a child go through something that terrified her was much worse than the experience itself. But she also noted that procedures and education had improved so much in the last fifteen years that the results were much more acceptable.

My recovery was amazingly fast. I attribute most of this to the wonderful family I came home to and all the support from Mom and Dad, brothers and sisters, and many wonderful neighbors. John and our four boys were all very helpful and wanted to do everything for me. However, I think the thing that helped me most was the last thing the doctor said to me as I was leaving to go home. He told me to get dressed as soon as I got home; if I laid around in pajamas, I would think I was sick, and I wasn't. Psychologically, this simple statement worked wonders. People would come to visit, and, because I was dressed and had my makeup on, they would tell me how great I looked—and that's how I began to feel.

Four days later we returned to the doctor's office to have the drains removed. It would be the first time I would see the scars. For a split second, I wondered if I really wanted John to see everything right then, but I decided that he had been through as much as I had and he deserved to be there. As they unwrapped the bandages, I was a little scared. I didn't know if *I* wanted to see what was left. But as all was revealed, John said, "You look great! It really looks good." God bless that wonderful man! And he was right. It did look good. I was still round and soft, and even though there were scars starting at the middle of my chest and traveling on both sides to my armpits, they were not ugly.

There were steristrips all across my chest, and approximately fifty staples were removed. The incisions were completely numb, so I felt nothing when the doctor removed the staples. However, the small incisions around the drain tubes were not numb, and it stung when they removed the drains. The doctor put saline in each implant. This created a tight feeling, although it didn't hurt. I had had an idea of what I would look like with the implants, and I was even more pleased than I had dreamed. It is so amazing to realize all that doctors can do to return things to normal. Fifteen years ago, my mother had to go through four separate surgeries, and she is still not happy with the results. My doctor, a very understanding, feeling person, was very concerned about helping me feel good about how I look.

It is now May 1990. I have had four appointments to have fluid added to the implants. I used to be small-breasted, but you would never know it now! It's great! I am almost forty years old, and there is no sagging. My breasts are firm but soft, and I never need to wear a bra again! I still do not have nipples, but I knew from the beginning that they would need to be removed to make sure all the tissue that might contain or eventually develop cancer was removed. There are some more steps that can be taken through minor surgery if I decide that I want to have reconstructed nipples. However, the lack of nipples doesn't bother me. My sister put it perfectly when she said, "You look just like a Barbie doll!"

As my doctor told me it would, this has given me a new perspective on life. Little problems don't seem so important anymore, and little happy things seem to mean so much. Everyday things that I might have ignored before now are worth taking time to notice and enjoy. Being home to enjoy Thanksgiving with all my family, sharing Christmas joys together, being there to see our second son receive his Eagle Scout award, sharing in each of my sons' birthdays, hugging them on Mother's Day—each of these events has an even more special meaning than it did before. I love life and the chance I have to live it. I am so grateful for the early detection of the cancer that allows me to be here to share the joy. My doctor said something to me that I will remember forever: "You will never again look at a beautiful sunset in quite the same way." And he is so right!

All in the Family, Part 2

John Glassey (Roxann's husband)

She lies sleeping, trying to shake off the effects of the anesthesia after her cancer surgery. What a beautiful woman. Intelligent, giving, so full of life for her boys and me.

We were married in 1971, blessed with four healthy, strong boys. It seemed that we would always be together. Our house would be paid for, I'd always have a new car, and we would never be in debt. Sometimes life has a cruel way of bringing you back from your dreams and placing you into reality.

It's 1974. She was a great mom. She married early and came to America in 1950 with Dad and three babies. They raised eight kids. I had a wonderful childhood, and, as it seems to most kids, I felt life would always go on with a mom and a dad.

It's June 1973. Mom is not feeling well; she says her bones ache. On July 4 that same year, I have a new son. My firstborn. Everyone wants to hold him. Mom holds him especially tight. She is very pleased but she seems weaker today. October 1973. Mom and Dad go to the doctor. They say she has bone cancer; however, they feel that it is caught in time. She's forty-five years old. With chemotherapy and much prayer, Mom seems better, or am I just hopeful? Who knows? July 1974. Mom is not doing well. Today she stays mostly in the bed Dad has made for her in the living room. I think he loves her more than he dares to express. He told me once that if he said his prayers, didn't do anything wrong, or step on any cracks, maybe she would be all right and recover fully from this vile cancer that has raped her body. I hope so, not just for me, but for him.

October 16, 1974. I've gone to work. The intercom calls me to the phone. It's Dad. MOM IS DEAD.

It's fifteen years later, 1989. There is something wrong with Roxy, my wife. Her mammogram. "Don't worry. It's probably just a bad picture. It happens all the time. Go ahead and go on the vacation you've planned. We can schedule a biopsy when you get back." So we go.

"We will have to take another picture; the last one seems to have some areas we need to look at." This is the fourth time that she has gone back. Something is terribly wrong. The technician won't tell us what is wrong. "You'll have to wait for the doctors to read the X-rays."

"We can't wait! My mother died of cancer. Her mother had a breast removed fifteen years ago from cancer. We can't wait." But we do.

They schedule the biopsy. We won't know the results for three days. So we wait again. After three days, we haven't heard, so she keeps calling the hospital. No answer. I have got to go to work.

The intercom calls me to the phone. It's Roxy. She's crying. "What? Please tell me."

"I have breast cancer."

All the fears come rushing back. It's 1974 again. Dear Lord, help me to be the husband that she deserves at this time. For the next few weeks, we cry together, and, although it's hard to explain, we seem to be growing even closer than before. Little things mean more to me. My family means more to me, but, most of all, Roxy means everything to me. I love her and want to be with her as much as I can. The cancer now has become ours. Selfish of me, maybe, but I feel that I am a part of her and she is a part of me. The doctor sits us down and talks to us. He feels that we have caught this cancer in time.

Roxy's aunt is diagnosed with breast cancer. She knew she had a lump, but she waited too long. It is probably terminal. Oh, please, Lord, don't let it happen to my Roxy!

We have had more time to think about things now and are almost rational. Roxy's left breast has invasive cancer, and her right breast is in question. The doctor has made many helpful suggestions as to what to do and we feel that we can make an educated decision now. We decide to have both breasts removed, a double mastectomy with reconstructive surgery performed directly after.

She's been in surgery for five hours. I'm not good at waiting; I've been waxing the van out in the parking lot. It's been seven hours now, and she's in recovery. I can see her through the window. The doctor says she came through the operation great. "We took out twenty-one nodes from the left side and four nodes from the right. They were all negative. We feel sure that we got it all. Well, 99 percent sure. No one gets 100 percent."

She's groggy from the anesthesia and needs to sleep. She is so beautiful, and I am so grateful.

We are six months out now. She has had one more reconstructive surgery, and things seem to be in order. I don't think I will ever pay for this house or drive a new car, and I do have a few more bills to pay. But life is good. I have four strong, healthy sons, a different outlook on things in general, and, by the grace of God, my beautiful wife, Roxy.

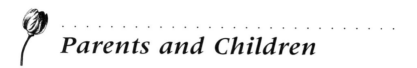

Parents and Children

Watching your child or your parent undergo the experience of breast cancer can be terrifying beyond words. The parents and children who wrote essays for this section often had a hard time verbalizing their anxiety and grief. The women themselves were better able to analyze their own reactions and those of their families.

In several cases, the women in this chapter are themselves children of parents who had suffered from or died of cancer—either breast cancer or some other type. Their family histories add an extra dimension of fear and courage to the challenge of facing their own diagnoses.

"It Isn't What Happens, It's What You Do About It" presents the author's determination to see her experience with cancer as a positive one, valuable to her own growth as a person and to the people she works with as a breast-cancer group leader. Her mother sincerely admires her daughter's attitude and ability to help others.

The author of "It Won't Happen to Me" recounts how she managed to cope with five children, a divorce, and financial survival while the experience of cancer and surgery kept happening again and again. Her daughter remembers what it was like to be eight years old and learn of her mother's cancer.

"To Question or Not to Question" is written by one of the few women whose breast cancer has known causes—radiation treatments for teenage acne. She stresses the way that cancer causes us to evaluate all aspects of our lives and to reprioritize. Her daughter explains how important it is for children to know what the disease is—and that it is not necessarily fatal—in order to handle what is happening to their mothers.

The final stories in this chapter were written by women whose parents suffered from cancer, one of them with fatal results. In "Breathing Life," the author had to overcome not only the shock of her diagnosis but also the grief and fear left over from her mother's death from breast cancer. She discusses the increasing numbers of breast-cancer patients, the lack of well-funded research, the need for education and for research money, and the odd priorities of a society that spends billions on weaponry and very little on efforts to save women's lives.

The author of "The Importance of Attitude" credits her own mother as a role model for how to handle the crisis of breast cancer. She also stresses the importance of getting accurate information about the disease and its treatments and of having realistic expectations about reconstruction.

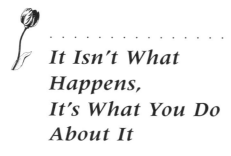

It Isn't What Happens, It's What You Do About It

Missy Cannell

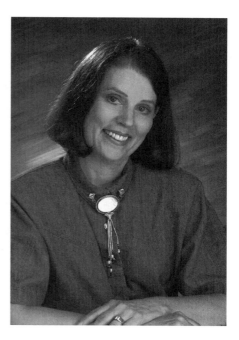

Missy says we all have life crises. Breast cancer has been her biggest. She was determined to make it a positive experience. She says her belief system determines her quality of life. She thinks illnesses come to us so we will look at our lives and change our beliefs, diet, habits, whatever it takes to get our bodies back on track. She thinks we are what we eat, what we think, and what we do.

Missy spends her time counseling breast-cancer patients, working in support groups, and generally cheering on the world. She is fifty years old, has two grown sons, and has been married to Joe for thirty years. They work together in an Italian restaurant they started fourteen years ago.

Medical Bio

Missy had had a twenty-year history of multiple breast cysts, with five biopsies and twenty-eight needle aspirations during that time period. So when a new lump appeared in the upper outer part of her right breast, she assumed that it was another cyst. She saw her doctor on the 17th of November, and a lump was noticed in the left breast as well. It was aspirated, and fluid was removed. When the lump in the right breast was aspirated, no fluid was retrieved, and because the lump was solid, a breast biopsy was recommended. On November 22, she had an outpatient breast biopsy, and the lump proved to be a breast cancer.

Missy elected to proceed with a radical mastectomy on the right, with a simple mastectomy on the left to obviate against the development of cancer in that breast. She also wanted the left breast removed because of her long history of difficult fibrocystic symptoms, the frequency of breast lumps, and the history of multiple cysts. Her breasts were extremely dense on the mammogram, so if a breast cancer did develop, it would be very difficult to detect.

Plans were made for the mastectomies to be followed by immediate reconstruction. However, during surgery, problems were encountered that made it best to delay reconstruction. There was no evidence of breast cancer in any of her lymph nodes.

Most people have a life crisis and then make changes. In my case, I started the self-improvement before the crisis. Then, when it happened, I felt completely prepared to deal with it and use it as a springboard for the rest of my life. I think having breast cancer gave me a chance to look at my life and fix the things that needed fixing. Here's how it happened.

One morning, sometime after turning forty, I was eating my second doughnut and enjoying the peacefulness of the moment. The two boys were off to school. My husband, Joe, was on his way to work at our restaurant. I happened to catch a glimpse of my changing figure—that over-forty, all-the-sand-in-the-hourglass-has-gone-to-the-bottom look. What a strange shape for someone who had always been skinny. I guess the combination of quitting smoking and the metabolism change that comes with age was catching up with me, and for the first time in my life, I looked fat. Hating that image and recalling a promise to Joe (made when I weighed ninety-five pounds) that I would always keep trim, I took a step that would change my life forever.

Joe had just changed his membership at the gym to a family plan so the boys could enjoy it; I thought there might be something there for me. I asked the boys if they thought I could do Nautilus, and they laughed and said, "Anyone can do Nautilus," so I made an appointment for instruction. This was the beginning of a new self-awareness for me. I promised myself if I started a workout program, it would be forever. So it was off to the gym three or four times a week, and it wasn't more than a month before I noticed some incredible changes. I was hooked. So much for the fat-housewife look.

Once I started seeing some results, I was really excited and changed my eating habits—no more doughnuts and lots more fruit and veggies. I also expanded my workout program to include the stationary bike, Stairmaster, and Versa-climber. I loved to walk with my friends and did that a lot, too.

But the very best thing I did was get my first bicycle when I was forty-two years old. It had hand brakes and skinny tires and was quite a change from the last bike I rode, which stopped when I pedaled backwards. I was really nervous about riding the bicycle with the skinny tires, so I would walk it across the street to a parking lot and practice shifting and braking. One day I saw a bike with fat tires, like the ones we rode as kids, and asked about it. It was a mountain bike, and I had to have one, so I traded in the skinny tires. My first ride was five-and-a-half miles up a canyon, and I almost died. I had to stop a lot, and I sweated a lot; but I made it, and it felt great.

In addition to exercise, I started reading. It seemed like a good balance to work on the inside as well as the outside. I began with biographies—Shelly Winters, Lauren Bacall, Joan Rivers, and Betty Ford. I lost the Betty Ford book before her breast surgery was described, and I can remember thinking, "I guess I wasn't supposed to read about mastectomies." Reading and exercise put me at a mental and physical peak, so that when the breast cancer was diagnosed, I saw it as a challenge, a test of my coping skills and my belief in the mind/body connection.

. . . .
Nothing but trouble

I have thought about my breasts and what they have meant to me. From birth to twelve or thirteen years old, I didn't have any but wanted them. The first bra I owned I found in a garbage can on my way home from elementary school. Three of us spotted some bras hanging over the sides, so we each grabbed one and ran off, giggling. When we got far enough away, we looked to see what size we had. I was the only one with a small 32A, so I took it home and washed it and waited to grow into it. The funny thing is that the garbage can belonged to Joe's family, and this first bra had belonged to my future sister-in-law.

Even before my first biopsy, I had extremely sore breasts, and, because of this, they were never part of our lovemaking. As Joe says, I turned him into an "ass man." In addition to being sore, they were very small. How small were they? Well, I have a birthday card that says, "Let me tell you a joke that will knock your tits off." On the inside it says, "Oh, you've already heard it." I even bought a T-shirt that had two fried eggs on it. I think I hated my breasts because they hurt all the time, I kept getting lumps, and they were too small, according to society's expectations of the perfect body. It seemed like I couldn't wait to have breasts, and once I got them, they were nothing but trouble.

In my late twenties, after both boys were born, I found the first lump. I went to a doctor as quickly as I could. He referred me to a surgeon, and I had a biopsy the following week. The lump was benign, fibrocystic. It was the first of many.

It's strange to remember how routine these lumps became. The fear of cancer dissipated with each lump that proved to be benign. But in March 1988, I found blood in my bra, and this time I was really concerned. So I called my doctor, and he referred me to a surgeon. What a blessing to meet this wonderful man!

Over the phone, he explained that this was probably a benign intra-ductal papilloma. We did surgery; he was right, and I was relieved. In the follow-up visits, he taught me more than I thought I needed to know about precancerous cells. He even did an evaluation of my chances of ever getting cancer—only 15 percent, according to my family history and pathology. Of course, the cancer was there as we were discussing the fact that it probably wasn't.

Shortly after the nipple-discharge surgery, a customer and friend brought me a thirty-page story about Fanny Birney, a woman who, in 1811, had undergone a mastectomy after drinking a wine cordial laced with laudanum as her only anesthetic. I can remember having a hard time concentrating while reading it because, first, it was very graphic, and, second, I didn't ever plan on having a mastectomy (and, if I did, this probably wasn't the best resource for a potential patient). Being given this story was as strange as losing the Betty Ford book before reading about her mastectomy.

I had a follow-up visit in July 1988, and, of course, there were more lumps. The doctor did a couple of needle aspirations, but a new lump on the right side wouldn't respond. When it still didn't respond in November, we set up a biopsy.

We used a local anesthetic so I would be clearheaded for work. The surgery took less than an hour. I was draped, so I couldn't see, but I tried to watch in the doctor's glasses. It was kind of fun talking to everyone in surgery. Wait a minute—is that a look of concern in the doctor's eye? No, he's just doing his work. So out of surgery and back to Short Stay for the cup of coffee they had promised.

I hardly had time to sip it, because the doctor was there. He said, "Missy, it was cancer." I said, "So what now?" He said, "I mean it, Missy, it's serious." I asked, "Do you want me to cry? Tell me I'm going to die and I'll cry." He said, "You're not going to die." I said, "I'm not the lady who hasn't had a mammogram for nine years. I had surgery on the other side eight months ago. I've had four mammograms in four years and was examined by you four months ago. Surely we've caught this in time." He asked if he could call Joe, and I said, "No, thanks. Let's not ruin his day." He asked if Joe and I could come by his office that afternoon to discuss my options. We did, and the only one that made sense was a bilateral mastectomy with immediate reconstruction.

....
Things always work out

Surgery was scheduled for December 6, 1988. Being self-employed, the thought of missing work and finding someone to fill in seemed insurmountable. But it wasn't. One of the many things I've learned is that it always works out. Somehow things get done. That's a very important thing to know.

The surgery took about five-and-a-half hours, and my mother and my dear friend Jackie spent the entire day waiting. In the recovery room, I remember trying to see the clock. The doctor came in and said something about not being able to do the implants, but not to worry, as we'd do them later. I felt a sense of disappointment, but I knew if he'd opted not to do the procedure, there must be a good reason. He told me that everything else had gone well, and, in spite of the fact that I'd had a rough day, it wasn't nearly as rough as my mother's and Jackie's. So he wheeled me into the elevator and then into my room. I don't think it's every day that a surgeon is involved in this part of the procedure, but this particular man seemed to forget there are others around who will do that. He always makes you and your family feel that you are his only patient, a quality that puts him in a class by himself.

As I arrived in my room, I remember muttering something about being glad this had happened to me. I don't know if I meant me as opposed to my mom or Jackie, or if I had some insight as to how my life was going to improve as a result of this.

The next thing I remember is a phone call from my sister-in-law in Los Angeles. She was crying. I asked, "What's wrong?"

"I'm just so happy you're alive!" she said.

I think it's interesting how people react to cancer. There is definitely a stigma. I was always surprised when people thought I might not live, because I never even considered the possibility of not living. I believe this happened to me so that I could direct my life and so I could go on to help others who would face this situation in the future.

My recuperation was pretty smooth. I really thought that I would be back to the gym in three or four days. Wrong. It wasn't painful, but my chest felt like a Mack truck was parked on it. Sleeping was a problem because I had to stay on my back all night. I would move from room to room, trying to find a comfortable bed or couch. Sometimes I'd watch television. Nonetheless, I got enough sleep to regain some strength.

Joe helped me wash and dry my hair the night I came home from the hospital. He's a much better cook than hairdresser, but I was more than happy to have clean hair. The next day, Jackie called to see if I wanted to go to our restaurant for dinner. I was happy to get out of the house for a couple of hours.

My first day back to work was December 12, six days after surgery. I'm sure if we weren't self-employed, I would never have considered this, but there was no one else who could work. I remembered all those people who had offered their assistance and called one of them. Together, we made it through a lunchtime rush. I took the orders and the money, and she did all the drinks and lifting. At first I moved quite slowly, but then it was as if I flipped my switch to automatic pilot. A lesson here is that people mean it when they offer help, and all you have to do is ask.

The first time I looked at my flat chest was about a week or so after surgery. I was alone in my bedroom. It was time to remove the bandages and see the decision I was to live with. It's always a little uncomfortable to get the gauze and tape away from the incision, so I was being as gentle as I could. As I got closer to the unveiling, I took a deep breath and sat down in preparation for what I was about to see. At last. What a surprise. I thought I was flat before the surgery, but this was definitely prepubescent.

Once I felt comfortable with myself, I called Joe in to have a look. This is an important part of my story, because I believe that sharing with him from the beginning kept him involved in the experience. It also kept the dialogue open, and I never felt like hiding or being embarrassed. Anyway, I was really shocked at his response: "You don't look any different." This may sound a bit funny or callous, but from the look on his face and the love in his eyes, I knew it meant that our relationship was untouched by this. His response was exactly what I needed, to hear that I was loved for all the things I am, not the two things I am not.

Christmas brought Joey home from college and Mark and his girlfriend Kelly for a visit. Kelly was a very special person throughout my entire breast-cancer experience. Her mother died from breast cancer when she was in her early teens. She's the one who worked for me during my surgery. I can remember how hard it was to tell her that I had cancer. I will never forget her face, and I'm sure that a lot of my drive to survive was to show her that with early detection, you can have breast cancer and live.

. . . .

The challenge of chemotherapy

With the new year came the challenge of chemotherapy. Up until then the only thing I knew about it was that people who had to do it went bald and threw up. Some people seem to handle throwing up, but it wasn't something I wanted on my list of things to do. In fact, I haven't thrown up for twenty years.

The weekend before chemo started, I had dinner with some friends. Afterward, we went to a couple's house for coffee and dessert. I found out later that it was arranged so they could tell me how to get through chemotherapy. There was only one expert there (an expert is someone who has experienced it); the others just had horror stories about other people who had gone through it. The expert, whose experience had been several years earlier, asked when I was to start. I told her I had picked Monday because I believed I could go to work and keep so busy I wouldn't have time to think about it. She asked if I didn't think it would be better if I went after work in case I embarrassed myself at work. I told her I did that every day anyway and that I'd have to do it my way.

Then they all started telling me dreadful stories about how some people feel it entering their veins, or how they get sick immediately after or hours later, or how they lose their hair. I argued that I'd read a lot and believed that positive thoughts would help me. They argued back and shared many examples of people who didn't want to be sick but were anyway. Soon I could see this was a standoff and the only way they would understand was to show them.

When Joe and I left, I felt horrible. I was angry and hurt, and, worst of all, I was afraid that they were right. I kept reliving the conversation, and it still hurt, and I was still scared. Then it hit me! This was a chance to turn a negative situation into a positive one. I now had several new reasons not to throw up or go bald. The anger left once I felt I could channel it to work for me. I realized that they believed they were helping me. They helped me all right—now I couldn't get sick.

So many times, we just accept others' beliefs as fact, without questioning them. All medication has side effects, and sometimes we know about them, but often we don't. Most drugs list nausea and vomiting as possible side effects, but usually this doesn't happen. Chemo, on the other hand, has a reputation of causing everyone who experiences it to have side effects, so they often do. I was given a book called *Chemo Therapy and You,* and it was the worst thing I've ever read. It was full of all the bad things to expect. I decided that I would experience chemotherapy and arrive at my own belief about it.

This seemed like the perfect challenge to test my new beliefs. I meditated a bit (my version is as simple as talking to myself), and I did a lot of praying. I made the decision to stay above it. I looked within myself for strength and hoped it would be there.

Well, stay above it I did. My body did six months of chemo, but my mind did everything but—I worked, worked out, traveled, remodeled, worked in the yard. I don't think there had ever been a six-month period in my life when I accomplished as much as I did while on chemotherapy.

We traveled to Los Angeles, Flaming Gorge, Sun Valley, and Jackson Hole. I never missed a day of work during chemo, and I continued exercising three times a week for the entire six months. In fact, I have maintained that for the past six years.

I decided to remodel the kitchen, a project that I had been putting off until Joey graduated or the truck was paid for or twenty other reasons. Well, I had borrowed Nike's motto—"Just Do It"—and the time was now. I got a bid, and it was outrageous, so I became a general contractor. I also decided to redecorate our bedroom, and when I wasn't working on either of these projects, I was in the yard, pulling roots out of the lawn. I found that while I was digging in the dirt, I was digging into me, and I think I learned a lot about myself. I gave up many old beliefs and formed some new ones. I'm sure it was an orchestration of all the reading and the life experiences of the past six years. I felt in total control of myself and capable of anything.

Upon completion of chemotherapy, I had a new me with a fresh outlook on life—and a beautiful home and yard. I even think all my relationships were better. What a terrific way to end an experience that is usually believed to be devastating.

It wasn't entirely without side effects. A couple of problems that I'm still seeking solutions for are the hot flashes and dry vagina that are direct results of chemotherapy. I stopped having periods within a couple of months of starting treatments. I thought it was great, until the hot flashes started. They are an incredible physiological experience. They come from nowhere and have the worst timing. You can't control them, but I'm working on it. They're better than having periods.

I've recently read that one thing you can do for dry vagina is to remain sexually active. It's supposed to help maintain some of the natural lubricating abilities of the vagina and also creates a decline in the frequency of hot flashes.

One of the totally unexpected side effects came during the chemotherapy. I was at work and opened a letter from my insurance company. I was amazed to find a notice that, because of the claims for my cancer surgery, the premium would increase 100 percent. I couldn't believe it. After two more increases, I dropped the policy.

I've since had several phone calls from insurance salesmen. I always say, "Before you go on, I want you to know I've had breast cancer." They say, "You have yourself a good day, ya hear," or "Sorry to bother you." These are things that make me angry, but I keep reminding myself that being angry only bothers me. No one else suffers. I think anger is a necessary emotion, but I also think we all need to learn to let go of it or use it to accomplish positive things.

....
I'll die with my boobs on

I scheduled reconstruction for October 1989. The presurgery tests were done on Friday for a Monday-morning surgery. This was definitely a more upbeat occasion. The doctor came in, and we discussed important things such as size and how long the procedure would take, and he said he'd run to look at my X-ray films and be right back. Well, his assistant came in and asked me to come with her. I asked if there was anything wrong, and she said, "There are spots on your lungs." I felt like my knees would collapse, but I kept walking into the room where my doctor and the films with the spots were. There were two X-rays side by side—last year's and last Friday's. There were two spots, one on each side, and from the look on the doctor's face, I could tell this was pretty serious stuff.

He said he'd do whatever I wanted—cancel, go ahead with the surgery, postpone, whatever. I asked a few questions, like, "What will happen if it's cancer?" He told me they would either do more chemo or perhaps use a drug called Tamoxifen. I remember thinking that I wouldn't do chemo again, because if this had happened while I was on it, my belief in it was destroyed. I thought about the hassle of rescheduling at work and decided to go ahead with the surgery, saying something like, "What the hell, I'll die with my boobs on."

There was some pain and discomfort from this surgery. It hurts more to put them on than it does to take them off. And, of course, it was back to sleeping on my back. Because my arms couldn't be raised above my head, I had to wait a week before they could do a CT scan. What a long week it was! Monday finally came, and the CT scan showed that the spots were not metastatic cancer but inflammation. We don't know what caused them, but a couple of my theories are that the chemo caused them (I remember having a rattle in my lungs after the first two treatments) or that it may have been all the dust from the remodeling of my house. At any rate, inflammation was a great relief.

Thanksgiving and Christmas were just ahead, and I could look forward to both of them as extra special. I was cancer-free and feeling great. Joe and I decided to give each other a trip to Hawaii in February. We thought it would be a great way to celebrate our new life together and my new boobs.

In January, a local breast-care center and Nordstrom's cosponsored a seminar entitled "Life After Breast Cancer." I was asked to participate as a panelist and model. Of course, I thought the seminar was a great idea and was more than happy to be involved. I really felt a need to share my experiences as a way of increasing women's awareness of the importance of early detection of breast cancer.

As the seminar approached, there were meetings and fittings. At the first meeting, the organizers from Nordstrom asked what kind of clothes we could wear, and we said we could wear anything, from swimsuits to evening clothes. But no one wanted to wear a swimsuit, not even me. However, I thought it was very important for the women attending to see someone who had experienced breast cancer modeling a swimsuit, so I said I'd do it. I couldn't believe that I'd volunteered, but then, most of the past year had been pretty unbelievable.

The week before the seminar was a busy one. I didn't have much time to worry about being half-naked in front of an audience. I was asked to interview with a local newspaper. There was a taped conversation for a radio station and a couple of TV spots. After seeing Julia Roberts in *Pretty Woman,* I feel this week of my life was comparable to her shopping spree. This wasn't Rodeo Drive, but to this forty-seven-year old who had just kicked cancer, this was much better. After the seminar, I bought the swimsuit—not only for my trip but as a symbol of my breast-cancer experience. The trip was fantastic.

Since returning home, I have been involved in the creation of a support group held weekly. I am a co-facilitator and work with a social worker. There is substantial proof that women who belong to support groups live longer than those who do not. It is also helpful to keep a daily journal. Our goal is that we all become better than we were before.

I believe I got cancer because of my lack of coping skills and a temporary breakdown of my immune system. I also believe that recognizing and changing my ability to cope will keep me from having a recurrence. There are many ways to heal your life. One is to take control and get rid of the things that don't matter. Another is to obtain the best medical advice and care. And finally, you can take the time to know and love yourself.

I had read in *Pathfinders,* by Gail Sheehy, about the hostages in Iran and how the ones that endured their downtime best were the ones who used it as a time for personal growth. Now, before my experience, I didn't consciously say, "Oh, I'll do this like the hostages." It's only been since my experience, in wondering why I seemed able to turn it into a really positive experience, that some answers have surfaced. I never asked, "Why me?" when I had cancer, but I've sure asked, "Why me?" in considering my ability to enhance my life as a result of it. I've read many books about breast cancer, and they always mention anger and devastation. I truly was never angry. I know that it isn't what happens, it's what you do about it; devastation occurs if you have no control. The self-discipline that I had developed and my wonderful doctors educating me about cancer and giving me choices put me in control.

Hopefully, we can all learn to face who we are and what we think about ourselves. For example, am I pretty because six people think I am?

Are those six people any better at judging than I am? If I feel pretty, that is the only thing that matters. This is true in all aspects of self-awareness. Am I a good mother according to others' beliefs, or do I believe I'm a good mother?

The only way to be the best is to develop self-love. Only then can we be loving to others and accept love from others. One of my favorite sayings is, "If you work on yourself, the rest of your life falls into place."

Breast cancer is the best thing that has ever happened to me. It validated a lot of my beliefs and taught me a lot about myself—about my strengths and my purpose on this earth. It directed my life toward helping other women through their own breast-cancer experience. Most important, without this experience, I might never have taken the time to know myself, and it would have been my loss.

. . . .
The personal becomes political

Since writing this chapter in June 1990, some unbelievable things have happened to me as a direct result of having breast cancer.

Early in 1991, I was helping a local breast-care center plan the third Life After Breast Cancer seminar, and we invited Dan Quayle, then vice president, to visit the center. He agreed to come in July, and I was chosen to represent the volunteers and receive an award on their behalf. It was an honor, and I was very excited.

On July 23, Dan Quayle spoke to 100 people at the governor's mansion. Half of them were breast-cancer survivors. After Vice President Quayle spoke about his involvement with breast cancer, our governor presented the award to me. I shook the governor's hand and then the vice president's hand. He pulled me close and gave me a very sincere hug. It was an incredible surprise, and, of course, I loved it.

In the meantime, the Breast Care Center was planning a trip to Washington, D.C., in October, and I had the opportunity to go. All of us at the Breast Care Center worked for weeks getting letters signed and ready to take to Washington. The letters asked our president, senators, and congressmen to allocate more funds for breast-cancer research.

Our departure was heartwarming. There was a big crowd with placards and banners, and some of the ladies read their letters. There was TV coverage and a lot of excitement.

The trip was as much fun as I've ever had in my life. I only slept twenty hours in five nights. There was so much to see and so much to do. We worked at the American Cancer Society getting the letters ready. We marched on the Capitol—something I still can't believe I've done.

Through my personal experiences, I have learned that our mind-body connection and nutrition are things we can focus on when other treatments end and that we must see breast cancer as an opportunity to change lifestyles, attitudes, and beliefs that are harmful. We need to live in the now and not waste time with worry or guilt. I believe that healthy eating can build healthy bodies and minds. I believe in prioritizing. Don't sweat the small stuff—and it's all small stuff. In the overall scheme of things, people, love, nature, and God are all that matter, not squeezing the toothpaste or burning dinner or getting your own way.

Breasts are related to nurturing, and as women we are the primary nurturers. Most often we forget to nurture ourselves. On the way to Washington, the flight attendant was demonstrating the use of the oxygen mask, stressing the importance of the adult putting the mask on first and then assisting the child—a great example of caring for yourself first so you can better care for others.

I believe that the empowering act of quitting smoking and the self-discipline of regular exercise helped me through this cancer experience. Now, three years out, my focus is on sharing my experience, taking time for myself, and exploring nutrition so I can continue this healthy lifestyle for another fifty years.

A Mother's Viewpoint: A Daughter Named Missy

Elizabeth Hansen (Missy Cannell's mother)

Actually, we did not name her Missy. Her real name is Caira (pronounced kay-eyé-ra), after an aunt of mine who was a beautiful person in every way. Although my daughter inherited the wonderful characteristics of the original Caira, she never cared for the name, because no one could pronounce it properly. *Missy* was one of my nicknames as a child, and it seemed to fit my daughter perfectly.

When I was growing up, cancer was a taboo subject, discussed in hushed tones by the grown-ups. I think I was ten or eleven when I heard that an uncle of mine had died of stomach cancer. It has just been in recent years that cancer has been discussed more freely, and it should be. The more we know and understand it, the better it can be faced. So when I learned that Missy had breast cancer, I had mixed emotions. She had had a history of many breast lumps over a period of fifteen or more years.

We learned of it just before Thanksgiving in 1988. She had such an upbeat attitude that the whole family was buoyed up. Missy prepared Thanksgiving dinner, and we had a wonderful time, but in the back of my mind there was a twinge of something (guilt?), a feeling that I should be worrying. But I have known for many years that worry accomplishes nothing.

It was not until December 6, 1988, when she came up from surgery, that something inside of me seemed to collapse. I was a complete wreck, although I tried to hide it. I don't know how I made it through the holidays. Everything seemed an impossible task: cards, baking, presents, etc. Somehow I got through it, and then it was January and chemotherapy time.

Chemotherapy was another subject about which I knew little, other than the horror stories about side effects. Missy's doctor, the one who administered the chemotherapy, told her that many women choose to have theirs on Fridays so they can have the weekends to recover. Missy told him she would have hers on Monday and then go to work! A gutsy gal, right? And she did just that.

I used to go to the restaurant to check her face and eyes. Sometimes, she looked like Missy, but it was plain that some days were better than others.

I don't know where Missy came by her strength and optimism. She was an outgoing, fetching little girl, the youngest of three. Many of her report cards came with the message, "Missy talks too much!" Apparently, the talking has paid off, as she has appeared on TV and radio and has made videos and participated in seminars. She is so articulate and talks about it constantly, which in itself is good therapy. She is a great believer in the influence of the mind over the body, and I truly believe she has something there.

Missy has become very active in support groups. Her doctor sends frightened women to her. They come scared and weepy, but after Missy talks with them they leave ready to fight with all their might and with a brighter attitude. She spends time on the phone with many of them. Some she has never met, but she encourages them to join one of the groups and to attend seminars. This, too, is therapy for her.

My other children have not been tested as Missy has been, and I pray they never will be. But if so, they have their sister to look to for strength and courage.

It Won't Happen to Me

Karen J. Johnson

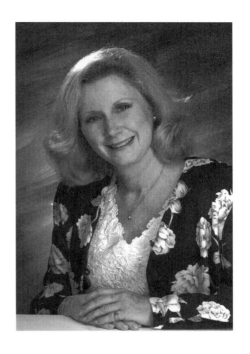

Karen was born and raised in the west, where she also attended college. She was married for seventeen years and has five children from that marriage. Karen has worked many jobs, sometimes seven at one time, to keep her family and home stable and allow her children their *various activities. She knows clearly where her priorities lie—with her children and grandchildren. Karen also enjoys cooking and baking, painting, skiing, gardening, and giving service to others. She has been the organizer, typist, and assistant editor of this book.*

Medical Bio

In February 1978, at the age of thirty, Karen discovered a lump in her right breast. A right breast biopsy confirmed that the mass was an infiltrating ductal carcinoma. She then underwent a right modified radical mastectomy. Three of twenty lymph nodes contained metastatic breast cancer. Two years later, she had right breast reconstruction and a left subcutaneous mastectomy with reconstruction.

Karen remained without evidence of recurrent breast cancer until January 1988, when a biopsy of her right chest wall revealed the presence of a poorly differentiated recurrent breast cancer. She then underwent radiation to her chest wall in addition to an experimental drug that shrinks tumors. Since then, she has demonstrated no further cancer recurrences.

Karen's reconstructive course has been complicated, and she has undergone multiple revisionary surgeries, including one episode of life-threatening toxic shock syndrome that was associated with a breast-implant infection.

Karen is living without evidence of recurrent disease, and after more than a dozen revisionary surgeries for reconstruction, she has finally obtained a stable and satisfactory reconstructive result.

The three-week-old baby had just settled down when I dashed for the shower. I found a marble-sized lump in my right breast, too prominent to be anything but trouble. Even though I was nursing my fifth child and had large breasts, this was still very noticeable. How could this be? They insist you do a breast self-examination when you leave the hospital. I had done mine and passed the test. That lump was not there three weeks ago; now it was there, and there was no denying it. A strange, uneasy feeling came over me, but at the same time, I was telling myself it was nothing, it couldn't be . . . after all, I was young, I had nursed all five children, I had no family history of cancer, and I was very healthy.

Early the next morning, I called a cancer specialist. My mother had raved about this doctor when he checked her fibrocystic tumors. His office said he would be glad to see me that day. After a thorough check, he felt it was a clogged milk duct and that it would be wisest to watch it for a month. At the end of the month, I went back. It was still there, and I was nervous. Something told me it was not right. I was still nursing my tiny baby. We made the decision to have a lumpectomy as an outpatient.

I was on the O.R. table, and, as they were about to give me anesthesia, a nurse said, "Quick, sign the consent form permitting us to perform a mastectomy if we need to."

"What is a mastectomy?" I asked.

There was a brief discussion, and I signed. I learned that if they found cancer, I would wake up without my breast; if both breasts were there, I was fine. Strange how this had not been discussed with me before.

In the recovery room, I raised both arms, and both breasts were there. The feeling of relief was great. I went home later that afternoon, slightly uncomfortable but happy.

The next day, I was still a little sore, and at 6:00 P.M. there was a phone call telling me that I had a fast-growing, rare breast cancer and that I had three hours to get to the hospital. They would be performing a modified radical mastectomy (whatever that meant) early in the morning.

It was hell. The fears. The worry of death. What would my husband think? Would I live long enough to raise my children? What about the six week old? Would I still be a woman? I had a nice figure, but what would I look like now?

Somewhere in the back of my mind, it was as if this weren't really happening to me, but, on the other hand, it was real. Such contradictions kept raging through my head!

That night in the hospital, my husband and I cried, talked, made plans for the children (just in case something happened), and tried to look for anything positive from this—that was the hard part. All in all, it was horrid, one of those moments that a person must go through to really understand.

The next morning, I had the modified radical mastectomy and felt like a truck loaded with cement had landed on my chest. They had forgotten to tell me about the numbness in my arm and the fact that I couldn't hold my baby or cuddle and hug my children. I could not even feed myself, let alone do such things as comb my hair, brush my teeth, etc. My ten-day stay in the hospital was one of mixed emotions, including a thankfulness that I was still alive.

After the ten days, the drain tubes, the dressings, the lack of movement in my arm, and the numbness, the pathology report came back indicating three out of twenty lymph nodes were involved. Damn! How does one go on? Is there anyone who really understands all of these questions in my heart and soul?

I think not!

I tried to take one day at a time. The love, support, cards, flowers, gifts, visits, and all the positive reinforcement helped me gain the courage to go on with a positive attitude. The surgeon did make my husband and me look at my disfigured chest on about the third day. It was shocking, but I am glad we looked together. I had been told there are women who never let their husbands see them—how sad for both parties. Both need to go through the hurting, as well as all of the other emotions this new disease creates.

On the tenth day, I went home. All the drain tubes were out, but the numb feeling had extended all the way to my elbow. Home and children were hard. I didn't feel well, but my emotions were all right. I was so busy keeping everyone else cheerful and helping them to understand, that I didn't really take time to adjust myself.

....
Pros and cons of prostheses

Going out in public, I was certain everyone knew about my chest, and I was positive they were looking at it. The only time I didn't care was six weeks after the surgery when I spoke at a cancer conference. The audience raved, and I felt then that I was handling everything fine. Airing my feelings in public helped me to understand myself better.

My aunt bought me some loose, baggy shirts and comfortable clothes that helped my self-esteem. I kept trying the little, soft, gift prosthesis that the cancer society had given me, but I was excited to shop for the real thing, because then no one would notice my chest (or so I thought).

I thought that if I went to the store for the prosthesis by myself, it would mean that I was doing fine mentally (funny how this sounds now, but then it seemed to be a good idea). The women were kind, but it was a frightful experience, and I should have had someone there with me. One should know better than to tackle mountains like this alone. The prosthesis was heavy and did not look natural and sometimes hurt, but I thought that it was a nice disguise.

Since they told me I would not regain complete use of my arm, I decided to take tennis lessons that summer (I was out to prove them wrong). It was hard, but was I proud of myself!

By the end of the summer, I had three more surgeries. When I first had the mastectomy, I was determined that I would never stoop so low as to have reconstructive surgery. I didn't want to be one of *those* kinds of women, those who make their breasts larger. And I also figured that if I had reconstruction, it would mean that I was not facing the fact that I had just had cancer. I wanted the world to know that I had faced it and that I was brave! I did not allow myself to cry much; after all, I felt that you either handled a major crisis like this or you didn't and ended up institutionalized. There was no gray area, no room for fluctuating, or so I thought. Who said you can't cry?

I was speaking more and more for women's groups and sharing my story. I would take numerous "Linda Lumpys" along for demonstrations, and, since I had purchased another prosthesis, I would also take my original large prosthesis. Once I remember opening the door to my van, and out spilled my demonstration box . . . artificial breasts all over! Yes, there were a variety of comments. Then there was the waterskiing incident. I was just learning to slalom and was on top of the clear, smooth-as-silk water when I felt a thudding against my chest. The prosthesis that I had pinned to my bathing suit had worked itself up and out of my suit and was beating against my chest. Well, there was nothing to do but take it off and throw it in the boat. That caused quite a few laughs.

I started to research the reconstruction idea. It wasn't just the waterskiing incident nor all the breasts falling out of my car (although that had an impact); it was also the fact that every night I would take off my clothes and put half of my chest on my dresser and take the other half to bed (how sexy can you feel?). I began to ask women how they felt after having reconstructive surgery. I couldn't imagine asking for more surgery; were they all crazy? But not one of the numerous women I asked ever regretted having reconstruction. I read everything I could get hold of and spoke to three doctors. I realized that I was missing out on something and that it would not mean that I was a dirty woman or mentally unstable.

I called a plastic surgeon and set the surgery date. I had a great result. Three months later (when the implant had settled into place), we finished the areola and nipple graft. At this time, because of numerous lumps and precancerous conditions, we decided to do a subcutaneous mastectomy on my left side, take off the nipple and areola, and put them back in their proper place. It sounds horrid, but it really was not as painful as the first modified radical mastectomy, and the recovery was fast. Best of all, the results were great!

Meanwhile, there were pains and lumps and tests and you-name-it. The surgeries started adding up, and, of course, I thought everything was cancer. Recurring tumors in the center of my chest, tubal ligation, salivary gland tumor, D & C's, liver biopsy, more D & C's, and finally a complete hysterectomy. I was three years out from the first taste of cancer when my husband of seventeen years decided to leave with the baby-sitter we had hired to help me. Now there were more mountains to climb and more challenges than I had ever dreamed possible. Five young children, no income, and only one way to look at this—with positive determination, tears, and by telling myself I could do anything. (I felt like the little engine that could.)

. . . .

Recurrence and radiation

Ten years from the first challenge of cancer, I had a recurrence of breast cancer (this time on the other side) and radiation therapy . . . more MOUNTAINS to climb! It seemed the doctors were a bit puzzled that I had gone so long in between major cancers.

My case was presented to the tumor boards of three local hospitals. The doctors did not have medical histories similar to mine in order to make a determination about treatment. No one could quite decide, so I did. I chose to have the radiation without standard chemotherapy, but I did take a tumor-shrinking drug.

I was so sick from the radiation that I promptly lost my job, some of my hair, most of my eyebrows, and all of my eyelashes. In March, when I finished the radiation, I remember attending a conference and feeling the room spin and my face feel hot and cold at the same time. I am not sure how

I drove myself home, but I remember pulling off the road several times to pass out before arriving home, ten miles away.

The burns on my side, chest, and throat were so bad that I had to prop my arm on pillows and cry. There seemed to be nothing I could do. I could not get free of the pain. It was hard to swallow because of the burns on my throat, lungs, and esophagus (my throat was so raw it would bleed all the time). I was educated about the effects of radiation, and everyone had told me it was easy compared to chemotherapy, but I was so sick. By September, I still had laryngitis, but I had slowly started to feel some strength—just in time for more surgery. The radiation had "cooked" my implant, and I was in terrific pain with the fluid filling my chest.

By January, I was ready for a new implant (how I hated all those months without one). I felt great until March when I awoke one night and thought I had the flu and passed out on the bathroom floor. By morning, I could not walk, and felt as though my strength was somehow being drained from my body. I am always surprised at how fast you can become so very ill. Of course, I landed in the hospital with an unknown infection and dehydration. In two days, I returned home for less than twenty-four hours. My daughter drove me back to the hospital, and that is where I stayed for ten days with a central line to my heart for the IVs that refused to stay in my arms and for the removal of my almost-new implant. I had developed cellulitis. The diagnosis? Strep in my blood. It wasn't just that I was the sickest I had ever been in my life, or that I had lost the implant, or that I was away from my children again, or that I had finals in my college classes—it is that I had just come the closest to death that I had ever come. I left the hospital with the central line into my heart for the home-IV antibiotics.

I still took my finals, including taking an algebra final in the hospital.

By August, I had another new implant. By the following January (1990), I had another tumor removed from my chest, and by July, I had my thirty-ninth surgery for the removal of what they thought to be two small tumors and to replace the implant again. They removed fifty-two tumors that were not malignant, and I think thirty-nine surgeries is definitely the number to stop at.

It's been one year since my last surgery. I feel good now. Sometimes I get more tired than I would like to, but all in all, I still keep up with my responsibilities, including working some part-time jobs.

Should we talk about the cost of forty-two surgeries, countless tests, scans, radiation, prescriptions, etc.? The closest figure I can come up with is over a quarter of a million dollars (after the insurance paid their part).

....
Reaching out

Life is always full of challenges. I am convinced that the secret of being successful and mentally safe is practicing positive thinking, believing in your affirmations, and believing that anything can be possible. I also believe in massive doses of love from family and close friends, along with some visualization that you can have or do or be anything you want. Given the many times I have been told that I had a short time to live, the many surgeries I have had, and the many odds I have beaten, there must be something to my way of thinking. Have I hurt? Have I feared death? Am I tired of pain and tired of worry? Am I sick of the financial burdens? Am I sick of the pain I see in my children's eyes? You'd better believe it!

But I choose to surround myself with the loved ones, the opportunities, and the knowledge that can help me through the challenges of cancer. I also choose to have the most positive attitude I can muster.

I could not have done it without my loving grandmother who reassured me, gave me unwavering love, and made me visualize that I could do anything if I was positive enough. My five beautiful children have always been right by my side, through laughter and tears, and have taken on many necessary roles. My sisters, parents, and friends have given me megadoses of support.

I should emphasize that the most important aspect of my experience was my early detection. If I had waited, I would not be alive today.

I was exposed to Reach to Recovery right away and begged to join their team. I attended the meetings and soon realized the value of the service they provided me and that I could provide to others. I started visiting other mastectomy patients. I tried to make a difference in their lives, and they always made a difference in mine. Eventually I took over as assistant director of Reach to Recovery. We made a TV commercial, had a fashion show, set up health fairs, and participated in many other public-awareness endeavors. I speak to church groups, business groups, and women's groups, among others. I have always benefited as much or more from the service I have given.

If you can get through the hurting, the valleys, the black clouds of this ugly illness, and somehow help someone else and still have love in your heart and hope for the future, then your agony will not have been in vain.

My family and I continue to have good attitudes and keep a bright hope for the future, despite the challenges that have crossed our path. I have met many new friends who help me visualize and do my affirmations. I am thankful for life!

Everyone is born with a gift.
If you are the cancer patient or the friend,
how well are you utilizing your gift?
My heartfelt thanks to everyone who has helped me realize mine,
and my heart goes out to anyone who is facing the black cloud of
cancer . . . NEVER give up!

. . . .

No Matter How Hard the Storm . . .

Tricia Paxton Warnock (Karen Johnson's daughter)

I have put off writing my story for so long. For some reason, it is much harder to write it down on paper than to talk about it.

I was eight years old when my best friend got cancer the first time. I don't remember all of the dates and specific events, but I will always remember the feelings and the fears I had when I was told Mom had cancer. Even now when she goes for check-ups or more exploratory surgery, there are fears.

I remember that first night so well. *Cancer*—what a scary word. Don't people die when they have cancer? I had never experienced the actual pain you get in your heart when you are so sad. I had never cried so much in my whole life and, at the time, thought I would never stop. I sat on Mom's lap and hugged her tight. Moms are not supposed to die, and I told her I wished it were me instead of her.

After that, it seemed like the days blurred into weeks. Being the oldest of five, I had to be strong. Ryan, the youngest in the family, was only three weeks old, so I quickly learned how to take care of the family. The experience of having so much responsibility is something I will never regret.

At the age of eight, the words *breast cancer* were not only scary but embarrassing. Everyone seemed to know about what happened, and when friends at school would ask about it, it was hard for me to say the word *breast*. They reacted with a lot of giggles and jokes. Many times I came home crying because of comments like, "Did your mom get her boob cut off?" It seemed that young people should know how to be more considerate, but maybe that was their way of dealing with a sensitive issue.

It was hard to think that everything could go back to normal, and, in a way, nothing did, but that does not mean we were not happy! I think when you are first faced with adversity, it is hard to look ahead and find hope and happiness, but it is there! I quickly learned many of the responsibilities that my mother had had. Now I appreciate the knowledge and experience I got by taking care of my newborn brother, cooking for the family, cleaning, and being a support to my brothers and sister.

Although there were many cancer-related surgeries during those years, Mom went ten years from the first cancer operation before the recurrence. Then during one of the suspicious exploratory surgeries, cancer again entered our busy lives. It was hard not to think it unfair. Hadn't Mom gone through enough? I was sure cancer would take her from us this time. She was very sick through twelve straight weeks of radiation therapy. One morning I went with her to a treatment. She wanted me to see and understand how the radiation worked. I cried as I watched her lie on a cold metal table as they "zapped" her chest with radiation.

This was part of another valuable experience. I am grateful that Mom was so open and honest about her cancer. Although some people think it may be better to keep the cancer experience hidden from their children, I don't believe it is. I appreciated her honesty and the time she took to explain everything. I felt that it helped me to accept and understand and work through the feelings and the emotions that I had.

As all of this was happening for the second time, I was seventeen years old and a senior in high school. Because I was older, this cancer brought new thoughts and concerns. My father had left after Mom had cancer the first time, so that put me in charge of the family. Now I was sure I would have to drop out of school to support everyone. But once again, after many months of sickness, Mom pulled ahead of the battle. I strongly believe her determination and will to live have kept her alive. Yes, we have had some trials to go through, but they have also come with many blessings.

One of the most important things that has come of this experience is that it has brought our family closer together and made us appreciate how blessed we are. We live for each moment; we cherish each day, each season, and each year. It is funny how such an experience brings out things that we should do anyway. We should not take for granted our lives, our health, and the special relationships we have.

Having a positive attitude and a strong faith in prayer, I know that no matter how hard the storm, there is always a rainbow.

To Question or Not to Question . . . That is the Question

Barbara Thayne Green

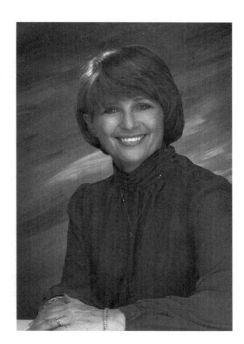

Firstborn of three daughters, Barbara attended college and was active in numerous organizations there. After a year of teaching elementary school, she married her childhood sweetheart and, from this marriage, two children were born, a son and a daughter. She continued to teach school. During the winter of her forty-second year, through a routine physical exam and ensuing mammogram, microcalcifications were discovered in her left breast tissue. No lump could be felt. She underwent tests, surgeries, bilateral mastectomies, and reconstructive surgeries. After about a year, her twenty-year marriage was dissolved. She is now remarried and is currently an elementary school principal.

Medical Bio

In January 1985, Barbara saw her primary-care physician for a routine breast examination. A screening mammogram demonstrated a cluster of small calcifications in her left breast, and a subsequent biopsy confirmed that these microcalcifications were associated with a small invasive ductal breast cancer. There were multiple areas of early breast cancer found in surrounding breast tissue.

When Barbara was a teenager, she had undergone radiation treatment to her back and chest to control acne problems. Therefore, a biopsy was done on her right breast, which also showed intraductal cancer.

Because radiation was thought to have played an important role in the development of Barbara's cancer, she was not a candidate for breast conservation. Mastectomy was elected as her best treatment option. She subsequently underwent a left modified radical mastectomy and a right simple mastectomy. None of Barbara's lymph nodes showed any evidence of metastatic spread.

She has been through multiple surgical procedures to obtain her prosthetic reconstructive results. At this time, she is living without evidence of recurrent disease.

Obediently, I unbuttoned my blouse and followed the shuffling, white-smocked, gray-haired man down the hall. Fourteen year olds do not question their elders. Do forty year olds? Should we just blindly obey those who claim to know what is best for us?

The X-ray machine was new. The treatment was new. The metal table was cold as I lay back, naked from the waist up—an embarrassing position for a fourteen-year-old female adolescent to be found in. But still I obeyed each direction given to me without question. The doctor placed protective lead pasties over my nipples and a lead blanket to protect me from the waist down. He left the room to seek protection from his new machine. I lay trustingly on the table, a young girl being cured of a slight case of adolescent acne by means of X-ray radiation, a young girl possibly being infected with a disease that would raise its ugly head twenty-five years later in the form of breast cancer.

You feel well. You look good. But inside is an insidious disease increasing exponentially in an attempt to eat up the good cells of your body.

You feel well. You look good. And a mammogram exposes an abnormality—microcalcifications. They might be an indicator of a malignancy.

You feel well. You look good. And your surgeon tells you he wants to amputate your breast.

You don't care how you look!

You want to feel well!

YOU WANT TO LIVE!

Do you question now? You question! You read! You get informed.

You have a biopsy. You confirm malignancy. You talk to your doctor for hours.

The most difficult time after diagnosis was the following week, a week of indecision, weighing options, facing my own mortality. Unexpected help and support surfaced through female acquaintances who, unbeknownst to me, had suffered and SURVIVED the same deadly diagnosis I had just received. The human mind receives subtle, unspoken messages when it sees a survivor: "She looks okay . . . I had no idea she was sick . . . She's alive . . . People do survive!" All these messages poured into a grateful mind and fueled the process of fighting to live.

These were better messages to fill my mind with than, "I'm too young to die . . . I want to take care of my children . . . I have so much left to do." But to turn these mournful thoughts into positive fighting action took the courage and belief I received from friends who had already fought the battle, from a doctor who spent hours educating me about my options, from a family who was constantly by my side, from a sister who left her teaching job in Colorado to care for me, and from a teaching colleague who spent her days teaching children and her nights teaching me.

She listened for hours as I talked and cried and tried to figure it all out, because that is the way I had always done things. I believed I controlled my world and could make everything work out the "right" way. It is difficult for a person like me to be out of control of what's happening in her life. God (or maybe a dermatologist several years before) had changed the game for me, and I had to function within this new set of rules.

It was also difficult for a person who had been so private about personal affairs to be suddenly thrust into the limelight and have the world know the most intimate things about her body. My mode of operation had always been to separate work, church, and home. But when the teacher, who also lives in the school community, takes an extended leave, everyone immediately knows why. Appearance had always been relatively important to me in that my work required me to be in front of many children and adults daily. Now I had to develop a sense of humor when people would greet me and obliquely drop their eyes down to my chest to try to determine what the surgeon's knife had left me with—or without!

Twice in the six weeks between mastectomy and reconstructive surgery, the artificial prosthesis, which outwardly gave my body great balance and shape, popped out of its assigned place in my brassiere and landed on the ground—once in a dressing room in a men's store and once on a main street downtown as I was getting out of my car.

This only made me more determined to go ahead with the reconstructive surgery that would make my body appear whole again. Now when I consider the fears a young woman must face when considering a mastectomy, I must stress the fact that if she chooses to have reconstructive surgery by a competent surgeon using the best available medical technology, life can continue with her body looking very much like it did before surgery.

Only upon the closest examination can my new breasts be determined to be different from the original pair. A fading, three-inch scar on the outside is the only telltale sign. Other than that, they look and feel very natural. I cannot wear a bikini, but I could not wear one before—it has nothing to do with the surgery.

Cancer became the impetus for many changes in my life. A marriage that had been in trouble for several years crumbled. When you face your own mortality, you realize that you may not have all the time in the world, so you bring to a conclusion things that are not working. You learn to say no when you are overprogrammed and cannot add one more thing. You learn to say yes to things you have been putting off until a better time. You learn to say "thank you" and "I love you" more often. You enjoy and appreciate the important things in life and eliminate the things that are not of value to you. You feel anger when told you should not get pregnant again because "the hormones could stir up cancer cells." Every time a new ache or pain appears, you remind yourself that your body is still allowed to have arthritis and other ordinary illnesses. You face the dating scene wondering whether or not your surgery will have an impact on serious relationships. You try to be up-front (pun intended) about it to allow the fainthearted to escape. You do not want someone around who cannot appreciate you for the whole person you now are. Life becomes richer. Instead of looking, you SEE; instead of being alive, you LIVE!

Looking back over the past five years, I realize the support I received from family, friends, and colleagues was unequivocally the most important aspect of my whole-person recovery. The doctors could heal my body, but my support network healed the rest of me. I also realize that had I eaten the whole cancer elephant in one sitting, I would not have survived. But by eating one bite at a time, I was able to take on all that I could handle until the next meal.

Talking with many people whose bodies have "experienced cancer," I have discovered the awareness of the disease is always with them, as it is with me. There is always the chance it could raise its ugly head again, but I am more aware of my body and the messages it gives me. I could also be hit by a Mack truck or be eaten by a shark while surfing at Malibu. I do not worry about the truck or the shark—or cancer. I choose now to live my life to its fullest. I choose not to squander a moment of the time I have with anything that is not important or valuable to me.

I always try to educate myself as to what is being done to and for me. To question or not to question? There is no question!

That Night I Dreamed of Death

Alisyn Thayne (Barbara Thayne Green's daughter)

It was a black night as my father and I crossed the busy street to enter the hospital. We reached the elevators and stepped inside. "Daddy, is Mom's room on the second floor?" I looked at his large face. He looked nervous, like he was about to do a tightrope act in a circus. He did not respond. "Daddy?" I gripped his hand even tighter.

"What? What did you say, honey?" Finally his face showed some signs of hearing me. "Nothing. Never mind."

When we reached her floor, we were greeted by a nurse who wore bright red lipstick. Some of it rubbed off onto her teeth, so when she smiled, she looked like a monkey with pink teeth.

"I'm sorry, sir. Children under sixteen are not allowed to pass this blue line." She pointed to the floor, where a thick blue line stretched from one wall to the other. My father released my hand and began talking to the nurse. "She has not seen her mother for a few days. Can you please make an exception? It is important!"

The nurse studied me with intent eyes. "Well, sir, I could get in trouble for this, but if you will only stay for a minute . . ." We were ushered down a busy hall full of bustling nurses.

My mother's room was at the end of the hallway. The nurse shut the door behind us. At first I could not see her face because of the dimness of the room, but finally everything came into focus, and then tears blurred my eyes. My mother was not the same. She seemed different. I could not describe how she was different; she just was. She was asleep. Her skin had sagged onto her cheekbones, and she looked so frail. My father held my shoulders as if to stop them from shaking. I was going to be brave because I was Mom's little helper.

I crept to the side of her bed and tried to get as close to her as the hospital bed would allow. It was not close enough. I could not hug her like I wanted to. Instead I whispered to her, hoping she could hear. "Mom? I am here now,

Mom, and I hope you are okay and come home soon and . . . I miss you." Dad was standing by the door ready to leave. I wasn't ready to leave her yet. We left anyway. That night I dreamed of death.

In the days my mom was gone, we tried to live like we always had. But things were not quite the same. My father tried to do everything right, but my brother and I knew it was different. At school I felt like I was being interviewed by thousands of people. "Where's your mom? What's she sick with?" She was a teacher at my school, so everyone knew and everyone gave me pitying looks.

I did not see my mother until a few days later when she finally came home. I came home from school expecting her to have the house back in order, but she was asleep on the couch and stayed that way for days.

After she returned, my grandparents, aunts and uncles, and other people were always at our home, either bringing food or just stopping to see how she was feeling. Each time the doorbell rang, she would greet visitors as if she were fully rested, even though she was tired and the previous visitor had just left ten minutes earlier. She was a strong person.

I liked to talk about the surgery. I understood the procedure; it had been explained to me in detail many times by my mom's doctor. I was often afraid, but family members were always helpful. The first time it really hit me that she had breast cancer was the day my aunt, my mom's best friend, and I were at the hospital as she was getting the bandages removed for the first time. My mother suggested that I leave the room, but the doctor asked me if I wanted to stay. I was curious, so I stayed and held tightly onto my aunt's hand and tried to keep my eyes open. Mother's eyes were gently closed, but her face had a tense expression. "Your mother is not going to look the same as she used to, Ali," the doctor explained. "Her chest will be missing tissue. It still may be very flat."

Everything the doctor said was true. Mom's usually full chest was as flat as a five-year-old's. It was strange. Her eyes sparkled from the tears as she tried to smile. "Well, this is certainly . . . different." I could tell it hurt her to see her body this way. It was comforting to know that she would not stay this way. Within four months, reconstructive surgery was performed, and things were the same as they had been before.

I will always remember the feeling I had as I was told that my mother had breast cancer: a fear that she might die. If the illness and the surgery had not been explained to me, I would not have felt so reassured that she was going to be okay. I think that all families need to talk about breast cancer so that everyone understands that breast cancer does not mean death. Nine years old at the time, I felt that if I ever got breast cancer, I would be fine. And now at the age of fifteen, I still feel the same way.

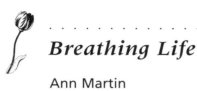

Breathing Life

Ann Martin

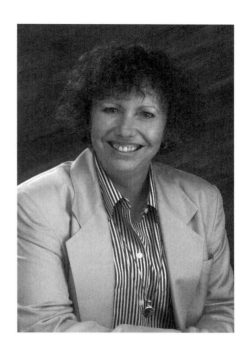

Ann ended her formal education as valedictorian of her high-school class but has continued educating herself by studying nature and pursuing classes throughout her career. Her focus is on writing and photography, and she has a profound interest in environmental issues and preservation, including habitats for our wildlife. She says, "I don't think I can be an effective writer if I fail to appreciate life by walking in its beauty." Ann is single and is the director of Medical Staff Services at a hospital.

Medical Bio

Ann's mother developed breast cancer at age thirty and eventually succumbed to the disease after developing a second primary breast cancer at age forty-eight. In addition, both of her mother's sisters died of breast cancer. Ann was intimately involved in caring for her mother and her aunts during the terminal phase of their breast cancers, and was very much aware of the significant risks she faced for developing breast cancer. So, while she was frightened, she was not surprised that the biopsy of a lump that developed in her right breast when she was thirty-three turned out to be a breast cancer. Ann underwent a right modified radical mastectomy in July 1981.

Ann's original breast cancer measured 1.5 centimeters, and none of her lymph nodes showed any evidence of metastatic disease. She was not treated with radiation or chemotherapy. She has been followed on a regular basis and has had no recurrent breast cancer. Because of persistent problems with scar tissue developing around her prostheses, she elected to have the breast implants removed in March 1990, after multiple attempts to correct the problem failed. She also elected to have a prophylactic simple mastectomy of the left breast. Ann is not contemplating any additional reconstructive surgery.

You didn't really know
why,
But suddenly it was time.
The surgeon's knife had
Done its best.

Time to think. A
Short straw. Long
Straws, too, but are
They long enough?

A leaf turned over
With a malignant
Thud, and suddenly
It was time to

Go on? Everyone said
Go on. I said go on.
Second life.

It was easy. One foot
In front of the other,
Breathing so my lungs
Barely knew.

Mother never told me there would be days like this, but none of us really knew then that the tendency for breast cancer extended throughout the female family tree. The darkest days of breast cancer were back in 1963, days my mother and two of her sisters knew only too well—days made darker because of archaic surgical techniques that made their breathing audible to the people in the room next door and maybe even the house next door. Dark days because they died.

A dark day came for me too, but there are infinite differences. I'm alive, and my breathing is barely heard and then only by me. My greatest task was (still is) overcoming the fear created by the intimate knowledge I had of the disease—I had watched it take my mother's life. But then she had watched it suck the last breath from my two aunts. My mother must have been terribly afraid. When I was told I probably had breast cancer, I began thinking of my mother's fear and my response, or lack of response, to it. Suddenly, in July 1981, when the final diagnosis came after an early morning lumpectomy, each and every thought piled fear upon fear. This is a story of fear turned round a bit.

There wasn't much difference between how I felt when they told me of my mother's disease and when they told me of mine. When the doctor said, "The lump was malignant; your mother has cancer," I felt paralyzed. I was sixteen years old, the youngest in the family, and the only child at home with a long-divorced mother. It is terrifying to know—or to think you know—that the most important person to you is going to die. She wanted to talk about her death, but I could not. The thought of her leaving was hard enough, and it seemed like talking out loud about her cancer made death even more imminent. The fear I felt at that time is impossible for me to describe, except to say it seemed never-ending, continuing even after her death five years later. I think the fear came from a loss of support in life and the recognition that our existence on this earth is so very flimsy. It was but another death, but it was my mother's death, and I did not truly face it until I had to face my own.

Her death was assumed because she was the third female sibling in her family to receive the diagnosis, and the other two were now represented by headstones in the cemetery. So in 1968, five years after her diagnosis, which had happened when the doom-filled loss of John Kennedy was still rich in our minds and my high school valedictory address was still a source of pride, my mother died and confirmed for me that breast cancer was indeed fatal. When my aunt died, I was sad; when my mother died, I was devastated.

It was during those years with her that pain took on a frigid depth, indifferent to medication or the hours on the clock. We both searched for understanding, but it was elusive, and we waited and cried. It was during those years when there was no support for women like her, and when her cries in the night blended with her breathing, that I became a person to be reckoned with. The promises of surefire cures in every magazine I picked up for five years added up and suddenly made me angry. My mother and I tried the ones we could afford, but most were not affordable to average people. I think people touting cures for terminal diseases are suspect. I think people touting relatively inaccessible cures for terminal diseases are contemptible. The mourning waned, but my resolve became more defined as I tallied the enormous cost of this disease to my existence—I had become a victim of breast cancer years before I developed it myself.

The years passed after my mother's death, and I gained some solace and resignation. I learned the architecture of my own breasts and performed the almost ritualistic examinations. Monthly palpation of my breasts was never easy for me. Even though I felt sure I would not find anything, always in the back of my mind was my mother, my aunts, and the fear of finding a lump. Although I thought about getting breast cancer and my future, I felt I was too young and the more serious worry would come after I was forty or so. Life was good and I was finally living it when a rather conspicuous lump reminded me not to get too comfortable.

During my self-examination the previous month, there had been something different—not a lump, but a difference in how it felt under my fingers. A month later, I felt the pronounced lump while toweling off after a swim. Then the needle aspiration reminded me that, even though I was just thirty-three years old, turning thirty-five was not a given. And the confirming biopsy reminded me of my aunts and my mother, and I was once again paralyzed. Painful memories flooded in, and it was difficult not to relive my mother's death with myself in the leading role. My physician, friends, and relatives kept talking and eventually made me believe that I was not my mother, that I could survive even though I would be the first in my family. Eventually I believed I would be the first in my family.

The decision to have surgery was not a difficult one for me, and on July 14, 1981, I underwent a modified radical mastectomy and lymph node resection. Loss of a breast cosmetically did not concern me—I wanted to survive the disease and felt an emotional need to have the more aggressive surgery. In retrospect, and speaking as a well person, I'm sure my survival would have been the same had I had the more conservative lumpectomy with radiation and lymph-node resection. Having lived with a mother who had undergone two radical mastectomies, I was pleasantly surprised when I viewed the right side of my chest for the first time. Of course, I thought my surgeon (and friend) had done an especially nice job, but truly all modifieds look good compared to the old radical, which spared nothing and extended up into the neck, over the rib cage, and down to the elbow.

During the days after my diagnosis, while I was wondering about my future, my niece (a wonderful, earthy, and caring spirit) called me with my astrological forecast. She said that the planet Uranus was impacting on something (I think it was my moon), causing terrible turmoil and uncertainty. She said that when Uranus does this, it feels as though you are being whirled around violently with no control. This definitely sounded like my astrological chart! However, after Uranus is done messing you up, it puts you down peacefully in a much better place than you were in before, or had ever been. I like Uranus, and I love my niece. And I love this new place, which has afforded me so much more knowledge and opportunity to feel things passionately, to remember, and to love. There is life after breast cancer. There is appreciation, almost spiritual, for all that is life. And there are the people, the people that you love and no longer take for granted.

I cannot remember the first time I noticed, but as time passed, it was as though I had been given new eyes. Not only did each day last longer, but the sunsets were prettier, the wildflowers were more plentiful and were mine to be with, the streams flowed for me to finally see, and books opened to pages that made me cry with the poetry of it all. I accepted my life anew and recognized the incredible opportunity it was. Some people just do that from the very start. I required a reminder.

I began to gain knowledge and recognize opportunities to speak out about our society's misplaced values. Much of my new knowledge was not pleasant, but I knew I would be remiss in not knowing it. I learned that each year the number of women dead from breast cancer continued to grow, no matter how I felt or what I did; I learned that the researchers could only do so much with limited funds and that what they had done was not nearly enough. The women who have died and are dying must wonder at the slow progress of research.

One in nine women will develop breast cancer,* and in spite of the research during the past thirty years, predominantly by the National Cancer Institute and the American Cancer Society, breast cancer continues as the number-one killer of women ages thirty to fifty. For women over fifty, it is second only to heart disease. Of the approximately 180,000 women who develop breast cancer this year, 45,000 will be beyond cure and will die from it.

These 45,000 women teach us about love and the alarming brevity of our lives. But they are eulogized only in churches and in the greeting-card section of stores, especially the Mother's Day cards, which eloquently describe women as not only the mainstay of families but of society as well, giving

....
*The current (1996) statistic is that one in eight women will have breast cancer.

solace and care and love. Mother's Day cards credit women with giving and sustaining life and for lighting the world. This credit does not seem to translate into value when research dollars are allocated. The only fitting eulogy now is to bring them out of obscurity and spend, spend, spend until the statistics are arrested and diminished.

One wonders if these women would be more valued if they were dying on battlefields sanctioned by our political leaders. Would we be more inclined to beef up defenses if these women were being killed by a menace attacking our shores? You may say it is not a realistic comparison, and it may not be completely realistic, in part because in the last thirty years many *more* women have died from breast cancer than men have died in battle. But it demonstrates what may and may not be noticed in this country. And the epidemic responsible for such losses is an invasion deserving of an equal response. Instead, we continue to hear about the rising statistics with no notable change in the level of research commitment.

There is also an alarming lack of consistency in the analysis of statistics. This confusion further illustrates where a waste of medical-scientific energies is occurring. Some feel that the incidence of breast cancer and mortality rates are increasing on paper, due merely to more sophisticated devices of diagnosing and tracking statistics, and some feel that the increase is real and alarming and may be due to environmental factors. The bottom line and dreadful truth is that more women are getting breast cancer than ever before. We know that women over fifty survive the disease no longer than they did twenty years ago, and women under fifty had a 5 percent greater mortality rate in 1985 than in 1975.[1] Even to a layperson, this illustrates the lack of substantive progress in thirty years of fighting breast cancer. Until this true and devastating loss is recognized for the catastrophe it is, women will continue to be held hostage to breast cancer, knowing that early detection is their only curative hope. And we still do not know how early is early enough. We who have been treated for breast cancer wait with aches and pains that scare us a bit but paralyze us completely if they come in the night. We live harder and wait and know that each day without a recurrence gives us hope that our early was early enough.

More research is needed, in part because of continued uncertainty about family history, diet, and estrogen replacement therapy as risk factors, and about the most effective means of treatment. Research must focus on developing tests for earlier detection, because even with knowledge about risk factors, we can only discover breast cancer after it has been present for several years. There continues to be much controversy in the medical and research community on how research funds should be spent.

As this controversy goes on, treatment of women who have breast cancer varies as well. There is justifiable concern relative to the benefits of chemotherapy and its harm to the body; and opinions about aggressive chemotherapy versus conservative, or any, chemotherapy at all differ among areas of the country and physicians. A report published by the General Accounting Office in January 1989 states that more than one-third of American women who should be getting chemotherapy are not.[2] Side effects apparently play an important role in some clinical decisions against aggressive chemotherapy, whereas other clinicians feel that profound side effects are part of the potentially lifesaving treatment. What are women to believe? *More* did not turn out to be *better* with mastectomies. But is more indeed better with chemotherapy? It may be hard to convince a breast-cancer patient with lymph-node involvement who knows the statistics for survival that chemotherapy may be more toxic than the cancer. The patient, of course, should be informed enough to take part in this decision and may want information from more than one oncologist. After all, it is her life, or death. But obviously, further research in these areas would greatly clarify the decisions she must face.

Long-standing research results indicate there are factors that may place an individual at higher risk for developing breast cancer. This research is valuable, as it increases awareness and improves our chances for the earliest possible detection. In my case, I was able to move toward a regime of breast self-examination and awareness, which may have saved my life. I met all the high-risk factors that I know of for breast cancer: maternal and aunt history, premenopausal and nulliparous (no children), and menstruation at an early age. We know what studies have shown about risk factors, but many women at very low risk develop breast cancer. *All women* must practice self-examination on a monthly basis.

Current research in oncogenes (aberrant cancer genes that appear in tumors) as well as in prevention of the disease is promising.[3] But is it enough? Is this country committing enough funds to prevention, therapies, and cures? A four-year cost estimate of the production of F-16s is approximately 15 billion dollars. Twenty-one nuclear submarines equipped with 899 nuclear missiles will cost 155 billion.[4] A billion here and a billion there thrown into research and into increasing accessibility to mammography seems a small price to pay if a dent is made in this disaster striking down our women. One may think me crazy comparing the defense of this country to the saving of women's lives. Must I be crazy to think these lives are more important than one more plane or one more submarine? It is time to emphatically wage war on breast cancer.

In 1989, 750 million dollars was appropriated for research on AIDS, while 77 million was allocated for research on breast cancer. We can all agree on the horror of AIDS, but AIDS has killed about 54,000 people since 1980. An incredible 430,000 women have died of breast cancer since 1980. Largely because of effective lobbying efforts by victims and potential victims, our government has allocated approximately ten times the money for research into a largely preventable disease that has killed about one-eighth the number of people as breast cancer. AIDS was recently called an epidemic; breast cancer has been an epidemic for twenty years. Why the disparity in funding? Perhaps it is fear on the part of the men who allocate such funds and not enough exposure to the rampant tragedy of breast cancer. We should be willing to lobby and to write letters to influential politicians. The sad truth remains that without a change in this nation's priorities, at least 45,000 women each year will continue to go to their graves.

There is much good news, though. I now believe that all things are possible, that a cure will eventually come. I remember and am grateful for the kindness of time, for knowing the women I have known, and even for being a victim of breast cancer. It gave me life, even though I feared it would give me death. It gave me new eyes that saw from side to side as well as in the distance. And at night, when tears form in my eyes for no real reason, I am grateful for this new weakness and wonder sometimes who I used to be. As for all the pain and fear, there are moments when there are none; but mostly, not a day goes by that I don't think about breast cancer and what a sledgehammer impact it has had on my life. But even with that, I'm not sure I would choose to avoid this experience, even if given the choice. For those 45,000 women annually who gain this knowledge and then take it elsewhere, I continue to weep—because selfishly, I would have liked so very much to have kept my loved one around longer. Wouldn't all of us?

A goldfish died today, and I was helpless to ease its way. It swam upside down and thrust its gills in and out, searching desperately for life. Once again, I thought of breast cancer, my mother, and how lucky I am to be alive.

. . . .
Notes

[1]"Anguish, Mystery and Hope," *New York Times Magazine,* April 23, 1988. This information is available elsewhere as well.

[2] Ibid.

[3] Ibid.

[4] The information relative to Trident submarines and the cost of F-16s is from *Aviation Week* and *Space Technology* magazines and the *Bulletin of the Atomic Scientists.*

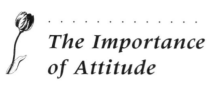

The Importance of Attitude

Dian Mahin

Dian and her husband travel extensively in the United States to celebrate their retirement. Prior to retirement, Dian worked as a nurse. When she is not traveling, Dian is committed to her volunteer work. She enjoys her three children and nine grandchildren, and describes herself as "people-oriented."

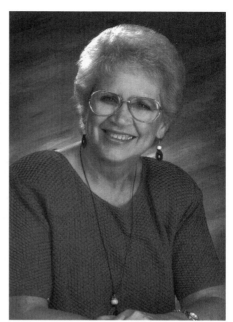

Medical Bio

Because Dian had a family history of breast cancer, she did regular breast self-examinations. In April 1978, she noticed a lump in her right breast. Her surgeon confirmed the presence of a movable but irregular mass in the upper outer quadrant of her right breast. A mammogram demonstrated a nodular mass suspicious for breast cancer.

A biopsy proved the lump to be a 2-centimeter infiltrating ductal carcinoma. She underwent a right modified radical mastectomy on May 8, 1978. She had a delayed reconstruction in July of the same year. She has also had a left simple mastectomy with reconstruction. Except for some problems with her reconstructive implants, which required additional revisionary surgery, Dian has remained well and has never had any symptoms or findings of recurrent breast cancer.

Fortunately for me, time has dimmed the memory of having had breast cancer. I can honestly say that now when I'm in front of a full-length mirror, I focus only on the lumps and bumps that have developed below my waist, never on the scars above my waist.

I vividly remember, however, a day in 1978 when, at the age of forty-one, I blundered upon a lump in my breast. It was a very busy time in my life and difficult to find time to see a doctor. My mother had experienced breast cancer several years before, and I knew that I must make time.

When my mother had breast cancer, she was sixty-five years old, a widow, and, to our knowledge, the first in our family to be stricken with this disease. I'm not sure that there was a lot of information available in 1962 regarding early detection, breast self-examination, mammography, or family history. The only information my sister and I received after our mother's surgery was when her doctor told us that we had better be careful because breast cancer ran in families—"the human family." We interpreted this as merely a feeble attempt to make a joke. Nevertheless, when I found a lump in my breast, I did know enough to see a doctor without delay.

I watched my mother go through a radical mastectomy without a tear, at least so far as I know. She was a very stalwart lady. She didn't have chemotherapy or radiation, so I assume now that she had no positive lymph nodes. She did what she had to do and got on with her life with not a lot of discussion about her fears. She passed away five years later of an unrelated illness.

I feel that my mother was an excellent role model for me. It had always appeared to me that she had breezed through her experience with breast cancer, and it never occurred to me to do otherwise. I was not afraid; I did what I had to do and got on with my life. I know that hers was not a breeze, nor was mine, but I believe that our attitude made it ever so much easier.

I saw the doctor on the Monday following my daughter's wedding. The lump was fairly large, and when he was unable to aspirate any fluid, he expressed to me his concern that it might be cancer. He scheduled me for several tests, which were accomplished that week, and I entered the hospital the following Monday.

I don't remember being terribly frightened, even though the odds were that it was cancer. In 1978 there were fewer options than there are now, so I knew that if it was cancer, I had no choice but a mastectomy. However, if I were given a choice today between lumpectomy and mastectomy, I would still choose mastectomy. A modified radical mastectomy such as mine does not leave you with the mutilation my mother suffered at the time of her surgery. For me, there is a sense of security in knowing that the cancerous breast was entirely removed. I would not want to rely on radiation if there turned out to be more cancer there than we knew.

Fortunately, there were no positive lymph nodes, and I was able to begin the healing process and look forward to reconstruction. I remember feeling that if I had to, I could live without a breast. My mother had a radical mastectomy, and I certainly looked much better than she had. I cried the first time I saw myself, but I've never been sure if it was shock at the way I looked or because they also removed the drain at that time, and it hurt! At any rate, those were the only tears, and I was very anxious to get on with my busy life.

My most negative feelings came after the reconstruction. I believe that I thought after surgery I would look the same as before, and I didn't. When I expressed my concerns to my doctor, he said, "Hey, you've had breast cancer, and you will never look the same again." That brought me back to reality, and, from then on, I was able to accept the changes in my body. At the time of reconstruction, they did a subcutaneous mastectomy on the opposite side and have attempted since then to make both sides more symmetrical. I have had a total of five surgeries: the mastectomy, two reconstructions, and two biopsies, which were both benign. I am able to accept the way I look with no problem. I can only say that I am very glad to be alive!

I developed breast cancer about the time that all the publicity began in all the magazines. I took a magazine with an article about breast cancer with me to the hospital, and when I went back for reconstruction, I had one with an article about that. I soon learned that the information you read in magazines may not be accurate and can be quite upsetting, so I stopped reading them and presented any questions I had to my doctor. I found that he did not agree with most of what I had read, and I liked what I heard from him much more. He had access to accurate information and was able to present it to me in a way that was easy to understand and easier to accept than the way it was usually presented in the magazines I had been reading. I was fortunate to have a doctor I could talk to, who was willing to take the time that I needed, and in whom I had complete trust.

Three years after my mastectomy, my marriage ended, and there were those who assumed that was why. Not so! My husband was very supportive for the most part, but there were other, unresolvable problems present long before that time. I was single for three years and then remarried, and I can honestly say that my having had breast cancer and a mastectomy has never been an issue, either with my former husband or with my current spouse. I am still the same person that I was before, and I still have two breasts, although they do now have more scars. I believe that *my* attitude is what makes the difference. Perhaps if I were less secure about my breasts it would affect my husband's attitude as well. I know he loves me, and so far as I'm concerned, my breasts have nothing to do with that.

Since my surgery, I have become a real breast-cancer crusader. I want to talk to and help educate anyone who is willing to listen. I was fortunate to work for my surgeon for a while and to be able to work closely with other women with breast cancer. I so enjoyed the association with those women, and even though my job was to help them, they were a tremendous help to me. To see the courage with which most of them faced this very frightening diagnosis was always an inspiration to me.

I believe that attitude plays a big part in recovering from any illness, and I am so grateful that my mother displayed to me a good attitude when she had breast cancer. I think that to maintain a good attitude you have to stay positive. I found that there are always those who want to share with you horror stories about someone they knew who didn't have a particularly good experience or outcome. I chose to disassociate myself from those kinds of people and spend my time with people who were more positive, who were willing to let me talk about my experience and my fears, and who were not uncomfortable when I did. There were always those who appeared very uncomfortable if the subject of my having breast cancer was raised. I found myself needing to talk about it sometimes and appreciated those who were willing to listen to me now and then.

I have two daughters, and I am aware of their risks. They are adults now and are very well educated about the risks. I will make sure that they do everything possible for early detection, and if, God forbid, it happens to them, I hope that they will be able to maintain a good attitude. I firmly believe that this is the best possible way to find the courage to accept those things that you cannot change.

Friends and Families

Having someone to talk to about the realities of breast cancer, particularly someone who cares about her, can greatly influence the way a woman handles the experience. As the authors of these stories testify, often the greatest sources of support for women with breast cancer are siblings, close friends, and other cancer patients.

The author of "Don't Sweat the Small Stuff" was blessed with a family hot line that swung into action at the news of the diagnosis and a group of friends that performed major surgery on her yard while she was in the hospital.

In "A Merry-go-round without an 'Off' Switch," the author expresses her frustration when family members who supported her often could not relate to her feelings and actions, and tells how she found that support through personal friends and a breast-cancer support group. The author of "Life and Breast" found comradeship and support from the group of patients who waited together for radiation-therapy treatments.

"A Month in the Life" is a diary written as the author was undergoing diagnosis and surgery. It captures the intensity, uncertainty, fear, and courage with which all of us begin our journey into the realm of cancer and the importance of a circle of friends to help us on that journey.

Finally, "Restoring Perspective" examines support from the point of view of one who gives it every day as a nurse-practitioner for a breast-care surgeon.

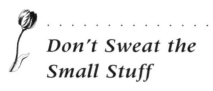

Don't Sweat the Small Stuff

Bridget Feighan

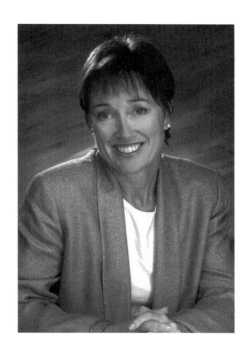

Bridget completed her master's degree in educational administration, including a certificate in special education, resource. She is currently the principal of a comprehensive special-education program for middle- and high-school students with behavioral disorders.

Bridget and her first husband, Bruce, were divorced in 1987. She met her current husband, Jeff, on a rafting trip. She loves long-distance bicycle touring, white-water river rafting, and swimming. She is also an avid cross-country skier and cross-country cyclist.

Medical Bio

In 1984, at the age of thirty-two, Bridget was on a river trip in Colorado when she noticed changes in the lump that she felt had been present in her breast for several years. It was now firmer and larger than she remembered it. Upon returning from her trip, she had a breast examination. The physician identified a 3-centimeter mass in her right breast. A biopsy confirmed a 3-centimeter infiltrating ductal cancer of the breast. After considerable consultation, Bridget elected to proceed with breast conservation treatment and underwent a reexcision of the biopsy site and an axillary lymphadenectomy. No evidence of breast cancer was identified in her lymph nodes. She then completed radiation therapy, which she tolerated without difficulty. She is currently well and without evidence of recurrent disease. She did not receive chemotherapy.

"You are a candidate for conservation therapy," my surgeon explained.

I had no idea how truly remarkable this news would turn out to be! A few days earlier, I had been diagnosed with breast cancer; my concern at the time was for my life—not for the loss of my breast. Fortunately I had taken enough time to deal with the idea of cancer first, so I then felt prepared to consider treatment options. I received enough information within ten days to make decisions about my breast cancer—decisions that would affect the rest of my life.

Conservation therapy is the preservation of the breast. It involves the combination of lumpectomy, total lymphadenectomy, and radiation therapy. A lumpectomy is the surgical removal of the section of breast that contains the malignant tumor. The lumpectomy is performed in conjunction with a total lymphadenectomy of the affected armpit. The lymph nodes are surgically removed to check for the possible spread of cancer. Radiation therapy eliminates any undetected cells that remain. If the cancer is small and detected early, conservation therapy is a considered option. The advantages of this procedure are that the majority of the breast is left intact and the loss of muscle strength and arm swelling are unlikely to occur. This treatment option is as effective in stopping the spread of cancer as other mastectomy procedures in cases similar to mine.

I was relaxing on a river-rafting trip through the Gates of Lodore in Colorado in June 1984. During the year, I worked as a teacher of emotionally handicapped adolescents, and I looked forward to my three months of vacation every summer. I routinely completed breast self-exams because I have fibrocystic disease. My frequent breast changes and lumps required persistent monitoring, and I was the only one who would recognize something unusual. On this particular trip, I noticed a breast lump that had not changed since my previous menstrual cycle. I remember thinking about it for the remaining days in this remote area and making a mental note to have it checked. When I returned home, I made an appointment with my physician. After completing a thorough breast exam, she recommended a mammogram the following day. The mammogram revealed a small mass in the right breast that looked suspiciously like cancer.

My sister, a local head nurse in labor and delivery, was the first person I called. She began a fevered search for information on breast cancer and on the recommended surgeons in the area. I felt quite dazed and grateful that she had the energy and knowledge to obtain this data. We picked up very useful information at the local office of the American Cancer Society and had information on treatment options for breast cancer mailed to my home. My physician recommended a surgeon, and we were able to visit with him the following day.

The surgeon reported that the characteristics of my lump as revealed by mammography indicated a breast biopsy needed to be completed. The surgeon said he felt "90 percent sure it was cancer." My sister Maureen sort of choked, and, as I watched her, the reality of my situation sank in. The surgeon was extremely straightforward and held out little hope that the tumor would turn out to be benign. I remember sarcastically saying to Maureen as we left his office, "Just give it to me straight and stop mincing words, doctor!" For a moment the laughter relieved our fears.

My husband returned from an out-of-town trip the following day. We talked about the cancer and the biopsy. It was very painful to discuss because we were both so afraid of the outcome. My husband was so worried during the entire ordeal that at the completion of my surgery, he began to have serious migraine headaches. The headaches incapacitated him to the point that he often had to go straight to bed. At times he was unable to accompany me to radiation treatments because of the severity of the headaches. He must have kept it all bottled up until I was home from the hospital. Then his level of anxiety about the cancer just pushed to the surface.

We talked about a mastectomy and agreed that we would do whatever was necessary. The biopsy was performed the following day, the lump excised, and the cancer confirmed. I found myself at home with my right breast bandaged and the news of cancer to accept on the same day. Maureen and I decided it was time to send in the Feighan forces (my family) and convey the bad news to my parents and sisters. Maureen began all the long-distance phone calls, because I knew my parents and sisters would want to make arrangements to visit. I remember feeling hazy from the anesthesia and overwhelmed by the pace of the day's events.

I strongly recommend securing a second medical opinion when you are faced with the decisions that cancer presents. I am so thankful that Maureen and I had obtained the information we had on cancer and on the recommended surgeons specializing in cancer of the breast. I was immediately able to establish a rapport with the second surgeon and found the answers to so many of my questions. My mother had been able to fly in by this time, and the office visits with the surgeon involved my mother, sister, husband, and me. Because my cancer was small and had been detected early, there were some alternative treatment options for my breast cancer. I know

now that the hours the surgeon spent with my family explaining procedures and answering questions were crucial for my confidence in approaching surgery.

During the ten days between my biopsy and eventual surgery, I was quite busy. I needed a bone scan, chest X-ray, and liver-functions tests. The surgeon explained that these tests were necessary to check if the disease had spread systemically to any parts of the body. This was a possibility I had not given much thought to, so waiting for results was very difficult. The surgeon did not want to recommend any procedures until he knew the extent of the cancer. The three days of waiting for results proved hardest for my mother. She was attending Catholic Mass daily, and my sisters depended on her long-distance phone calls to keep them informed. We really smoked the phone lines with what we now refer to as the "Feighan Hot Line"! My sisters waited patiently to make arrangements for their visits. My husband waited quietly and patiently, keeping everything inside.

There was no evidence of systemic disease and so the discussions of conservation therapy began. The lumpectomy would involve reexcision of the biopsy site to assure clear margins from the cancer. The total lymphadenec-tomy under the affected right arm would involve the removal of the lymph nodes for pathological examination. A course of radiation therapy for six to eight weeks would follow the surgical procedures. I realized that the river-rafting trips I had planned for the remainder of the summer would have to wait another year. This was not going to be the year I would finally float the Grand Canyon for twenty-one days.

I met with the radiotherapist, and my husband and I discussed the advantages and disadvantages of radiation therapy. Again I felt extremely lucky that I had the hospital facility so close to my home, since it would involve daily visits five days a week for six to eight weeks. We understood that conservation therapy demonstrated comparable survival rates to other treatments in which the breast is not preserved. If the cancer were to occur again at a later day, it would still be possible to have a mastectomy, if it were indicated. The disadvantages of the radiation therapy were discussed. The skin reaction to the treatments is similar to a sunburn and may require daily skin care. The radiation may affect the bone marrow where the blood cells are made, and this could limit the effectiveness of chemotherapy if it were needed later. The radiation therapy could also cause some scarring or atrophy of the breast.

My surgeon arranged for me to visit with a former patient, a Reach to Recovery volunteer, through the local chapter of the American Cancer Society. The woman was a nurse at a local hospital, and she spoke about her mastectomy. She explained that conservation therapy had not been an option in her particular case. In talking with her, I realized again how lucky I was to be considered a candidate for conservation therapy and to be able to keep my breast. I now had enough information to make a sound decision. I chose conservation therapy, and I have never regretted my decision. When dealing with the bad news of something like cancer, I feel it is important to take advantage of the good news—conservation therapy.

Dealing with cancer has changed my entire perspective on life. Regardless of the type of cancer or treatment options you have, I feel that your perspective on life will be altered. The entire cancer experience created more stress on Bruce and me than either of us were aware of at the time. I know at times I relied so heavily on my mother and sister that I unintentionally excluded Bruce. The cancer brought the issue of our indecision to have children to the foreground. The pathology reports revealed that my breast cancer was estrogen positive. This meant that my cancer was influenced by my estrogen level and that a pregnancy could place me at some risk for a recurrence.

My close friends, Bruce's family, and my family were at a loss to know what to do for me. They had all sent flowers, cards, and even meals, but still wanted to be more involved. My sister Maureen's husband, David, rose to the occasion. He organized the whole group while I was in the hospital for the three days. They replaced the field in my backyard with a fenced-in, sodded area complete with an underground sprinkling system. They even planted a wildflower garden using native plants. I returned to find the whole area transformed, and I was presented an album of pictures taken during the activity. The album remains one of my most prized possessions.

Some individuals view the rest of their lives as a cancer watch and anticipate a recurrence, but others use the experience to adopt what I call the don't-sweat-the-small-stuff perspective. The small stuff, such as daily disappointments and shortcomings, does not seem to matter in the grander scheme of things. The importance of your family and dear friends becomes clearly defined. At the completion of the summer, with my radiation therapy behind me, my husband and I had a grand party for our family and friends. It was the don't-sweat-the-small-stuff party, complete with our logo printed on our T-shirts. This was our opportunity to celebrate and say thanks.

My goal is to keep this perspective alive. I am now six years postcancer, and I make a conscious effort to maintain all I've learned about myself throughout this experience. I intend to remain cancer-free and to continue working with women diagnosed with cancer so they too can benefit from my experience.

A Merry-go-round without an "Off" Switch

Marie Carnesecca Knowles

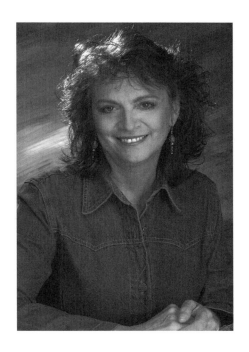

Marie attended Catholic schools as a girl and, more recently, has taken English classes at a local college as a step towards fulfilling her dream to write a novel. Marie has procrastinated putting together a keepsake book of her poems for her family and close friends. ("Hopefully the great feeling and therapy I gained while writing this chapter will propel me into action.") Several of Marie's poems have been published. She loves family skiing and crocheting in the winter warmth of her home.

Her children and grandchildren are her special loves. Marie is presently employed at a computer company.

Medical Bio

In June 1989, at the age of forty-four, Marie noted a lump in her right breast. Her examining physician confirmed a 2.5-centimeter lump and also identified a lump in her armpit. A mammogram showed additional suspicious findings. She then underwent a breast biopsy with the findings of a 2.5-centimeter breast cancer. She chose a modified radical mastectomy. Two of the eleven lymph nodes removed from her right armpit at the time of her mastectomy showed evidence of cancer. She then had courses of both standard adjuvant chemotherapy and radiation therapy. She has remained well, without evidence of recurrent breast cancer, and has undergone reconstruction.

In 1988, I read Jill Ireland's book about her ordeal with breast cancer. When I finished, I put the book on a shelf with relief, certain that I would never have to face the same disease. In 1989, I watched Ann Jillian's story on television about her episode with breast cancer. Again, relief.

Cancer was not a "me" disease, but it did belong to other people. I had educated myself about breast cancer; I had had mammograms every two years since turning thirty-five. But I just did not fit the breast cancer mold. I started my periods when I was twelve and had my first child when I was nineteen and my last at twenty-four. Most importantly, I had no family history of breast cancer. I was safe!

. . . .
"We cannot be certain . . ."

On June 23, 1989, at 8:00 A.M., I was putting on my bra, and I felt a definite lump on the areola. By 9:15 A.M., I was sitting in front of my gynecologist. The doctor had given me a complete physical three months earlier; there was no lump at that time. (My next regular mammogram would have been scheduled for the following September, two years from my last one.) After examining me, he sent me down the hall and into the hospital for an immediate mammogram. He did his best to reassure me and told me to have the radiologist call him with the results.

The mammogram showed an abnormal cyst or mammary gland, but the radiologist seemed optimistic about what he saw. He scheduled me for an ultrasound because he needed to look even closer at the evidence. He tried to aspirate the lump with a needle but was only able to get a few drops of liquid on the needle's tip. He took it to the pathologist and came back to say that they were optimistic about everything so far. But he did add, looking me square in the eyes, "We cannot be certain. It is an abnormal lump and must be removed and biopsied." He thought the lump seemed smaller than before he had inserted the needle into it. Then he rattled off something long and Latin-sounding that I did not understand but was willing to accept, as I had his optimism. He asked me if I would like to talk to my doctor, so while still on the ultrasound table, I spoke to my doctor on the telephone after the radiologist had told her what he had found. He tried again to reassure me.

"It is Friday!" I yelled. "I want action and answers. Please do not make me wait over the weekend. Take the lump out now," I pleaded. But the radiologist made my appointment for Monday morning. I went home to wait.

I could not keep my fingers off that lump. I began to work the breast tissue between my fingers. It felt hard and solid, unlike my left breast, which felt soft and movable. And my fingers, in their search for reassurance, came across a large, egg-shaped lump between my right breast and my underarm. I froze. My husband, Bill, tried to calm my frantic reaction to this newfound fear. My uneasiness grew, and my imagination ran miles ahead of me.

Finally, Monday morning. The surgeon was optimistic about the mammogram pictures she had looked at earlier that day in the hospital. I showed her the swollen node I had discovered a few days before. "Why didn't my doctor or the radiologist notice a lump this large?" I asked her. "And if they did, why didn't they tell me about it?"

"Well," she responded, "actually both doctors mentioned the lump to me but felt there was no need to alarm you any more than they already had." That infuriated me, and my mood was not too hot anyway. I told her that was unfair: "It is my body, and I have the right to know every little thing about it." This outburst from me was unusual, but, all of a sudden, when it came down to cancer's potential to push and shove, I wanted full ownership of my body parts. No cancer was going to push and shove me anywhere. From then on, I was very adamant about what doctors could and could not do to me, especially when it came to anything that had to do with breast cancer.

The doctor told me that both lumps would have to be removed and biopsied. The morning of the biopsy, I tried to be brave, but all I could do was cry. I was emotionally exhausted. My husband tried to console me. "You are giving up before you know the outcome." But I was not; I was just plain scared.

The sharp needle pricks numbed my breast and alerted my senses to an even higher degree. The doctor removed the tumor, which I asked to see. I could tell the doctor felt positive about the outcome. She deadened the swollen node but said, "We will not cut this yet, because if the quick-freeze biopsy comes back as malignant, we will remove all of your lymph nodes in that area during the surgery you choose."

The telephone in the operating room rang. My mind froze. The surgeon said a few words on the telephone, rushed back to my side, and looked me square in the eyes. I wanted to reach up and rewrite the words that I saw in her eyes even before they came from her lips. "It is a cancer, Marie." They ripped through my gut like a bullet seeking its target. My blood pressure exited the monitor. Shock waves rippled through me. Everything happened so swiftly after that.

....
In a matter of minutes, I had become my own family history

My life was changed in so few hours. My husband was brought into a small recovery room to see me and my surgeon. My mother and sisters were still in the waiting room and had no idea that something was not right. When my husband came through the door, his face looked questioningly at both the doctor and me. The words rolled off my tongue in what felt like slow motion. "It is cancer, Bill." I cannot remember what his face looked like, but I felt his shock and fear penetrate me and add to my own.

The doctor immediately spilled my options on the table. I had decisions to make. For some reason, I felt totally in control. I knew instantly that I wanted the breast removed. All I could think of was to get this mound of cancer off my body and get it off now. I found myself pleading with her to take me back into the operating room and get it all over with. She said that was impossible because I needed to have blood work done and a chest X-ray. She had to be certain that the cancer had not spread to other vital organs.

That was terrifying to hear, because the possibility of more cancer had not occurred to me. Another dimension of fear piled on top of the deadly pile I was already gathering. To top it off, I would have to wait until Wednesday for the results of these tests I felt could mean life or death for me.

Finally, frozen with fear, I watched my mother's and my two sisters' reactions as they came into that little room and I had to say the word that I could not believe I was saying. *Cancer.* "It is cancer," I cried.

My daughter arrived within minutes. She had already encountered her father, who was on the telephone in the waiting room as she came through the door. They had cried together before she was brought to see me. My heart ached most for her. She begged me to tell her she was only dreaming. "It is real, Michelle," I cried. "We have to face it. We cannot even wish it away." I held her and we cried together. I felt like I was holding her as a baby again. And oh, how I instantly longed to be back in those days when living seemed easy and my children were babies and toddlers. I began to feel anger for what I could not touch from the past and for what I could not change for now and for my future. I wanted to go back one week in time and start living it over again so the results would be different.

The actual modified radical mastectomy was scheduled for June 29, 1989, six days after I had discovered the lump. And again, I went home to wait. Upon leaving the hospital, my sisters asked me what I wanted to do. I said that I wanted everyone with me, my sons and my daughter-in-law, and all of my nieces and nephews and brothers. I wanted my whole, large family to surround me with life. I wanted to feel safe in the arms of my family's love and support.

Going home was not the same and never would be again. I knew I was going to die. Many tears were shed as each family member arrived. I sobbed uncontrollably when my second son, Kelly, arrived with his girlfriend Brooke, and when Leticia, my daughter-in-law, finally arrived from work. My oldest son, Lee, was out of town on business. I longed to hold him to me with my other children, needing desperately to console and protect them from what I had brought into all of our lives.

As darkness descended that long, awful day, I became afraid of the dark for the first time in my life. An eerie feeling began to seep through me. I wanted life and light to stay with me forever. The darkness seemed to be a sign of my own life light flickering out.

. . . .

My guardian angel goes to work

I went to bed still clutched by fear. I felt the presence of my father, who had died nine years earlier, and my brother, who had died of leukemia at the age of three, just a couple of months before my birth. I had always felt that I knew him somehow. I believe that he and I met as we traveled on our separate journeys, his to death and mine to life. Now I lay in bed with cancer, his disease, and I was frightened that he and my father had come for me. But a quiet calmness settled over me, and I knew that they were only there to bring me comfort. When they drifted away that night, they left me with the guardian angel I had known as a child but forgotten as an adult. She stays by my side constantly, and she taught me how to say my night prayers again. My father and brother had brought me the gifts of prayer and hope. I already possessed the gift of a very strong faith in God, and many times during the past year I have prayed and begged him for the strength to make it through certain days when the going seemed to have no end, and fear wanted to swallow me whole.

On Wednesday, I was relieved to learn that the tests done the day before showed no sign of cancer in other areas of my body. But I was extremely let down when the pathology report came back the day after my surgery. I held my breath when the doctor came into my room. "Let me have it," I said to her. And she did! "You have two nodes that were positive. One was large and metastasized; the other was very small and barely affected." The doctor said she felt good because my cancer was estrogen positive, and that was a good sign.

I recovered fast from the mastectomy. My theory is that I had to get up and be well. Staying down and sick was just too risky, too much like being dead. So I got up to live, and nothing was going to stop me.

I remained in a numbed and shocked condition for the six-week recovery. The response of friends and acquaintances was overwhelming; the stream of flowers, cards, books, and telephone calls was never ending. At that time, I began to sense a feeling of such concern for my well-being from so many people that it heightened my sense of concern for myself. But I lived pretty calmly through those weeks, and the diagnosis and reality became obscure. The thought of death grew distant.

. . . .

The chemotherapy bitch

I had coped pretty well until the morning of my first treatment. Then I literally lost it. I freaked out to the point at which it felt like my hair was standing on end. It was the thought of the word *chemotherapy* as much as anything else. Even today, two months after finishing chemotherapy, I still shiver at the thought of it. Chemotherapy revealed the reality of what I was up against. The concern that everyone had shown hit me like a ten-ton truck. I was fighting for my life. That morning I felt the war begin within me.

My husband tried to convince me that chemotherapy was my ally. I had to work hard to accept that. I made up my own little fight song, like I was a cheerleader in high school. I sang it constantly. "The bitch is chemotherapy, na-na-na-na-na, and she will eat my cancer cells, na-na-na-na-na, but she cannot have my hair'r'r, and she won't make me sick'r'r, na-na-na-na-na."

But she did.

She made me sick, and I could deal with that. But when her scraggly fingers pulled out my entire head of beautiful hair after only two injections, her greedy pleasures at my expense made me hate her. She was truly a bitch, even to the end. My coping skills went into the plastic bag with my hair. How was I supposed to cope with cancer when all of a sudden I was a bald woman who looked like a perfect stranger to me?

So here I was—a bald, one-breasted, sexually unattractive person who did not even recognize herself in the mirror. That mirror became my enemy.

My therapist and friend, Linda, suggested that when I look in the mirror, I should look directly into my eyes and search for myself there. That same evening, my husband said, "Your eyes are larger and prettier with no hair on your head, and they are you." So that is where I would find me, hidden inside myself like a frightened child peeking out from behind my eyes. I thought God must have decided that I was just not humble enough. In my reflection in the mirror, I saw myself on knees of humility.

Life for me through this period of time was like being on a merry-go-round without an "off" switch. It went 'round and 'round in circles, and I could not get off until the treatments ended. I did my chemotherapy over a one-year period. All of the other women I knew did theirs over a six-month period and were able to get on with their lives much more quickly than I was. But the large doses I had been taking to complete chemotherapy in six months were not leaving me with what I felt was any quality to my life. I made the difficult decision to take smaller doses and go for one year.

Being on chemotherapy that long began to really wear down my body. During the seventh month, my energy level would often drop to zero. I spent a great portion of every afternoon on my living-room couch. If I had a commitment for an evening that took me away from home, that afternoon body rest was a must. I folded up between 9:30 and 10:00 every evening, no matter where I was. My husband, without complaint, would lovingly get me home to bed. I firmly believed that I must rest my body to heal it.

. . . .
Mourning period

During this time, I was hit hard with the very personal loss of my breast. I grieved and mourned the loss of this most sensual piece of my sexuality. I was determined that the people I loved must accept the loss too. I would show my scar and boyish, flat chest to anyone willing to look. I watched my family turn away or cringe every time I would bare this truth to them or anyone else. My daughter, my son Kelly, and my daughter-in-law had the least difficulty looking at me and trying to accept the deformity with me. My husband and oldest son, Lee, seemed to want my blouses and nightgowns buttoned up to my chin. I knew that these negative reactions stemmed from the deep hurt my family felt for me and that my mother and my sisters could not bear to look at the nothingness that peered out from where a natural cleavage used to be.

The same reactions often came when I would bare my baldness to someone. These reactions hurt me deeply. I tried desperately to understand people and their actions, while, at the same time, I was fighting so hard to accept the gross and vile act my body had suffered. On the whole, however, I considered my family very supportive; they were then and still are my life sources, especially my husband and daughter, who lived under the same roof with me, and my younger sister, Tina, and her daughters, who spent some part of almost every day with me while I was in treatment. They saw firsthand every up and down time I had.

I was baffled about what my breasts had stood for. Sexuality was an important but small piece of this puzzle. Breasts were meant to sustain life, not to take it. I nourished my babies from the same breasts that had turned against me and could possibly cause my demise. What a cruel twist of fate.

The helpless feeling at having my health begin to fail at age forty-five was overwhelming. I felt so old and frail, and it had all happened so suddenly. I have written my obituary, which will probably have to be changed one day when I die old and gray and not from cancer at all.

. . . .

Life enhancement the hard way

I knew two things within seconds of hearing I had cancer. The first was that I had to thank God that my children were raised and had someone they loved to lean on for support when I died. I knew my husband could survive without me. The second was that I had to change the way I was living, eating, and coping. I had to take better care of myself than I had done the past few years. So my first thoughts were of death and the continuation of life entwined. Somehow, the survival instinct started to play its game with my mind at the same time that I was convinced that cancer meant death.

My friend Missy calls her breast cancer her life enhancer. I can say that my life this year has had many positive rewards that have occurred because of this nightmare. The greatest of these is an improved relationship with my husband. However, I do wish life had been able to enhance itself some other way.

My last four weeks of chemotherapy were very emotional. It shocked me that all of a sudden I was afraid to let go of this bitch who had been protecting me every week for one year. I would be going it on my own. My fear level peaked. In a one-week period, a friend and support-group member had a recurrence of breast cancer, this time in her lungs, which devastated me. I learned of recurrences in two young women I knew from another support group. But the most difficult event that week was the death from breast-cancer recurrence of a very special woman who had been an inspiration to me even before my own cancer brought reality too close for comfort. I have often thought that the fear these cases caused in me increased my power to fight this curse even harder.

It hurts so to watch people you care for have to live through the hell of recurrence. The first diagnosis is difficult enough. I can only try to imagine what it is like the second time around. Death must seem even more inevitable. My heart ached for each of these women, as it had at the news of Jill Ireland's death one month before. Her death hit me so hard. I felt like I had lost a very dear friend or family member. I tried to talk with my sisters about my feelings, but they could not understand why I was so affected by the death of someone I did not even know. I think Jill was a symbol of hope and optimism for all of us. I do not believe she lost her battle. She lost her life, but she was a winner because of her determination, courage, and joy in the life she lived, despite the battle she was fighting. She was a positive model to all of us as sisters who share in this disease that steals breasts and lives.

People tell me often that I am courageous and brave. They say they could not handle cancer as well as I have; but they really could. They would handle it because they would have no choice. If being brave and courageous is feeling insecure about my future, experiencing a fear of dying, and crying for what seems like no reason at all and often out of the blue, then I guess I am courageous and brave. But I feel cowardly at times. There are just those days that are difficult to get through, until the next day, when things seem better. My guess is, it will be like that for the rest of my precious life. Treatments end and life goes on, but knowing cancer can creep up on you once more is a thought that never really leaves you in total peace and harmony. I speak only for myself here. Each woman's reaction to her own breast-cancer experience is personal and individual.

I have learned to give and receive hugs; I have learned the importance of human touch. The cold and alone feelings that often overwhelmed me through this past year created a great need for the warmth of another living being. I believe that need opened up my ability to show more affection to the people I love and care about, including the women in my support groups. I try to hug my children more, and I am more verbal with the "I love you's." I have always had a hard time expressing these feelings. I was good at show-ing them in other ways, but it is the actual demonstration of these feelings that is becoming so rewarding.

I always wondered what people meant when they said to live one day at a time. Now I know and respect what each moment in a day stands for.

. . . .

Cancer and families

I have seen how my breast cancer affects my family not just physically but emotionally, especially my mother. I have made her greatest fear come true—that she might lose another child to the same disease. I have changed all of our lives. Living will never be taken for granted again.

Communication with my family concerning breast cancer is often diffi-cult when it comes to trying to share my fears and rewards with them. I have always been able to share my deepest and most intimate feelings with my sisters. The block that has come between us is very difficult for me, but I understand them. I think they must feel so helpless. That is where the support group I attend each week takes over. Only other women who have had this experience can truly understand me. All of the women I have met there have become a part of my life source.

Letting go of fear and realizing I must accept what I cannot change has been a process with many stages.

. . . .

Afterthoughts on expectations and realities

Looking back on chemotherapy and radiation treatments is difficult. I try to convince myself that The Year of Chemo was not so bad. The mixture of drugs and chemicals I had was not as strong as that given to women today their first time around. Knowing this makes me feel a little less safe and yet thankful, so my convictions are filled with doubts. My disdain at the thought of chemotherapy does not hinder my knowing that I feel safer because I did it.

I would give the cancer back—but with hesitancy; I cherish the friends I have gained because of breast cancer. I have also lost many to this disease and will lose many more, but the pain of losing is worth the joy of having known them.

Now when I am called to reach out to someone who is just beginning to live with this, I try to gently prepare them for what may lie ahead. I never say, "You will not lose your hair," or, "Chemo will probably not make you sick." I want to protect them in any way possible, but I remember my own experience, and I wish it had not been quite so sugarcoated with other people's optimism. I took to heart all of that positive advice and felt like a failure when I did not live up to any of it. The fact is, I did lose my hair quickly and I did get sick, and I learned fast that each person's experience is individual. No one should try to predict what might happen, including the oncologist.

We women with breast cancer expect so much of ourselves from the very beginning. Every book says you must be optimistic, you must always have a good attitude, you must image and meditate, and on and on. I felt so desperate to live that I overwhelmed myself by trying to do it all as fast and as often as I could. If I had a down day or I didn't complete a certain path of meditation or positive imaging, I was sure I was going to die; I wasn't living up to what became a chore of demanding expectations of myself. I now know there is time. Cancer can take lives quickly, but it does not kill you in a day. I finally came to a place of acceptance in my continued search for more knowledge about breast cancer, understanding that even if I suffered recurrence, I would not die tomorrow.

I have learned that there is time in between biopsy and actual surgery to do some investigating. There is not a desperate need to rush the whole horrifying experience into four or five days. I would still have chosen to have my breast removed because of the swollen nodes I found along with the lump, but I and many women today regret the rush encouraged by some of our surgeons. It is such a vulnerable time, and learning in an instant that you have cancer is so terrifying that most of us rely on whatever the doctor says at the moment. Knowledgeable doctors give their patients the information and time to make thoughtful decisions.

My guardian angel still entwines her golden rope with my determination to hold onto this life for as long as possible. Where she begins and where she ends, I do not know; she is always floating in my aura. I feel her protective wings flutter around me. She glitters with enthusiasm to light my way each day. I wonder if she will grow old with me or if she is immortal. Will she be given another to surround with faith and comfort when my days come to an end? Will she take me to that place of glory and white lights when I have reached total peace of mind again, her mission achieved? Am I to be a guardian angel? I wonder often how I will reach that place among the stars. Swiftly, I hope—oh so swiftly. As Euripedes wrote, "Who knows but life be that which men call death, and death what men call life?"

Breast Cancer
She haunts my optimism
and flaunts her ghostly figure
of reality at my days.
She lingers on horizons
in dreams, where hope sees her
as someone else.
Perhaps just a figment of my imagination.
My illusion is transparent.
Her off-white gowns
flutter in morning breezes.
And I whisper:
Don't come back
wearing gowns of black . . .

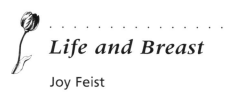

Life and Breast

Joy Feist

Joylene (Joy), a native of southern California, was an art major in college. In 1972 she founded her own company, Joy's Interior Design, Inc., which she continues to operate. Joy is married to Dan Feist and together they have raised four children (two from Joy's previous marriage). Joy is a superb amateur photographer: Kodak has awarded her five regional awards and 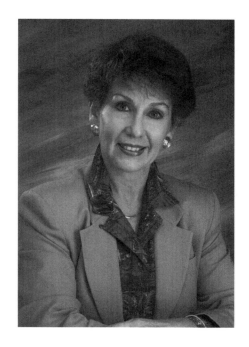 *one national award in the Kodak International Newspaper Snapshot Awards contest. Special projects include lecturing to various women's organizations concerning breast-cancer awareness, including early detection and prevention. She calls her program, "Taking Charge of Your Body—What You Don't Know Can Kill You."*

Medical Bio

Joy was forty-three years old in 1988 when a routine mammogram revealed a lump in her left breast. The lump proved to be a 2.4-centimeter infiltrating ductal breast cancer. Joy elected to be treated with breast conservation. The lumpectomy and removal of her lymph nodes was accomplished, and she was subsequently treated with radiation therapy. Her breast-cancer treatment also included a course of chemotherapy. Joy continues to be treated for a side effect known as lymphedema (swelling of the arm), a complication from the surgery that removed a sampling of lymph nodes necessary to stage the extent of her disease. To date, Joy has no evidence of breast-cancer recurrence.

I've yet to meet anyone old enough to remember the day President Kennedy was assassinated who couldn't tell me exactly what he or she was doing when the news came. Similarly, I've never met any cancer patients who couldn't tell me the details of their life at the moment they heard they had cancer. The course of life is changed forever; the big question is, "How long is forever?"

On November 29, 1988, at age forty-three, I found myself in this situation. The doctor called my office late one afternoon to report the results of a fine needle aspiration of a lump in my left breast. I had not found the lump myself; I wasn't even looking for it. My seventy-three-year-old mother thought she had a problem, and I accompanied her to the clinic where we both had mammograms, her first and my second.

I had heeded the advice of my gynecologist and had had a baseline mammogram when I turned forty. The advice I failed to heed was to return for subsequent mammograms at one- or two-year intervals. Now, three years later, because of my mother, who turned out to be just fine, I was back at the clinic having a second mammogram. It revealed a tumor large enough to have easily been felt if I had been performing a breast self-exam on a regular monthly basis.

The intrusion of breast cancer into my happy and satisfying life was a major shock. How could this be happening to such a healthy person with no bad habits—ever! There was no breast cancer in my mother or her ninety-four-year-old mother or her three full-breasted sisters and their daughters. (I have since learned that 70 percent of women diagnosed with breast cancer have no known risk factors.) I was aware that my breasts had fibrocystic tendencies, common to many women. However, I had decided not to drive myself and my doctor crazy with these routine breast changes—sound thinking as long as you do self-exams faithfully and check out any irregularities that persist longer than a few months. But I had been lulled into complacency through the years and neglected my routine. I went in for my yearly PAP tests without fail, and I thought that if there was a problem, my doctor would find it when he performed his own breast examination on me. Too bad I knew him so well that I distracted him with my yearly chitchat about who's doing what and where so-and-so is these days. My dad always taught me and my two brothers that accidents (auto) happen when two people are not paying attention. I wish I had extended this good advice to routine health care.

Faced with a diagnosis of breast cancer, I was suddenly enlightened as to what things in life are truly important and irreversible. The interior-design firm I had founded sixteen years earlier suddenly seemed way down on my list of priorities. Fortunately, I had responsible and loyal personnel in whom I could trust to carry on in my absence.

With the help of my wonderful family—my husband, Dan; my sons, Brent, Chad, David; and my daughter, Kimberly—I was determined to act responsibly, because I knew I was the one who would live or die with the consequences of this dreaded disease. Although scared beyond words, I knew I had better not feel sorry for myself because I had the family and the resources to sustain me. My heart went out to those women I met during the course of my treatment who didn't have what I had in the way of help and still managed—or, in some cases, didn't manage—the terrible burdens and challenges set upon them through no fault of their own.

. . . .
Exploring the options

When I was diagnosed, my husband was out of town, and when he called that night as usual, I delivered the bad news. He was stunned to hear the needle aspiration was positive, which meant for sure I did have the disease. Dan said he would catch the first flight home. As much as I wanted him to do that so I could have him comfort me, I knew he needed to complete his business in Los Angeles. I assured him I was okay, considering the circumstances, and would have more input for him after I met with my doctor in the morning.

I decided to educate myself and become an active partner in my treatment options. For example, the advice I received from the surgeon who eventually performed my surgery was to have a modified radical mastectomy (complete removal of the breast). Although there are many good reasons to relinquish a breast—first and foremost because it could save your life—there are also sound reasons for lesser surgery. I wanted to explore all my options before I gave up a breast.

I was surprised at the surgeon's suggestion because of things I had heard when Nancy Reagan had had her mastectomy a year or so before. She was a perfect candidate for the lesser surgery, but she chose a mastectomy. The American Cancer Society and the National Cancer Institute had both criticized her decision. They contended that as a high-profile person, she was setting a poor example in light of current studies showing mastectomy and lumpectomy patients having the same long-term survival rates. She later defended her decision, and then I understood. She said she was extremely small breasted in the first place. Secondly, she said, "Ronnie is a leg man." And finally, she said she didn't want six consecutive weeks of radiation therapy, which is a must for lumpectomy. (Radiation is needed to treat the site of the primary tumor after removal to ensure there are no cancer cells still at large.) The First Lady wanted a quick recovery so she could accompany the President on his historic trip to Russia to meet with Prime Minister Gorbachev.

I sought second and third opinions. The surgeon who had performed the needle aspiration was very helpful in setting up various appointments with other specialists in a timely manner. I appreciated my wishes being respected, but I was puzzled by her recommendation. This particular surgeon was female and close to my own age. Surely another woman would understand why I wanted to keep my breast if possible. Wasn't it the old stereotypical male doctor who found it hard to break with medical tradition? For a hundred years, breast-cancer treatment meant removal of the breast and everything else that could be cut out of the area.

I read everything I could find on the subject and interviewed other women. Anyone who wants to rush you to the hospital without time for personal research in an effort to get the cancer out of your body as soon as possible is wrong. The cancer has been there for a number of years already, and a few more weeks to ponder your course of action is essential to a satisfactory outcome, one you can live with for a long time to come. It's okay to ask detailed questions of doctors; the good ones welcome it and respect your inquiries. Find a doctor who will be your partner instead of your boss.

. . . .
'Tis the season for a lumpectomy

I wanted to have a lumpectomy, which removes the cancerous tumor and a margin of normal tissue surrounding it. I was a candidate for this lesser surgery because of the size, location, and other aspects of my particular tumor. Regardless of whether you have a lumpectomy or mastectomy, the surgeon must also do an axillary dissection—the removal of ten to twenty-five lymph nodes located in the armpit of the affected side. A pathologist then examines the tissue to determine whether or not the cancer has spread to any of the nodes. This is called staging.

It is quite possible that cancer cells from the primary tumor have escaped their location in the breast and traveled via the lymph system to the nodes in the underarm area. Cancer cells can also be transported by means of blood vessels to vital organs such as the lungs, liver, and bones. This is why node-positive women (those whose lymph nodes show cancerous cells) are recommended for chemotherapy in addition to surgery. However, node-negative women may also want to have chemotherapy. Such was my decision. My lymph nodes were negative, but nobody can assure me that cancer cells didn't find a blood vessel to invade and subsequently travel to my lungs, liver, or bones to set up housekeeping and eventually kill me. We probably all remember our mothers telling us to eat our spinach and drink our milk so we would have strong, healthy bodies. Whether our mothers knew it or not, they were really saying good nutrition boosts our immune systems. Our bodies could be combating cancer long before we know we have it.

December l, 1988, found me keeping an appointment with the radiologists who would present the conservation-treatment option and further evaluate my candidacy for the procedure. As I look back at my journal (which I began at age twelve), I am reminded of some of the emotions I experienced the day of my appointment. The weather was gorgeous, and I found myself noticing every little detail. There were snowy patches here and there, but the streets and sidewalks were clear. The sky was brilliantly blue with white, puffy clouds scattered about. The air was crisp and clean, and the sun was warm and comforting. As the car radio played Christmas carols, I felt I was hearing them for the very first time. I couldn't help but wonder if I would be around to hear carols next Christmas. When you are healthy and relatively young, you have the luxury of thinking about the future; I used to see a long line of days, months, and years beautifully stretched out in that wonderful word, *future*. It always gave me another day to get done what I didn't accomplish today. With tears rolling down my cheeks, I realized I had never fully appreciated the beauty of everyday life.

I met with the doctors at the radiation clinic. They were wonderful at answering my questions and detailing what I could expect from the radiation treatment that would follow a lumpectomy. I felt good about my decision to pursue the lumpectomy. As the senior radiologist answered my various questions, he drew illustrations on the paper that lined the examination table. At the end of our discussion, the paper looked like a surrealistic drawing by Salvador Dalî. I also checked out the reconstruction options from a plastic surgeon just to see what that would entail should I choose mastectomy with reconstruction. Because of my breast size, I was told my healthy right breast might have to be reduced in size to more closely match the reconstructed left side. All things considered, I felt the lumpectomy was my best option.

There was the possibility that once inside the breast, my surgeon would encounter other evidence of the disease, and our plan would have to change. For example, if she found other diseased areas, she would have to remove the entire breast. We called the possible actions plan A for simple lumpectomy and plan B for mastectomy.

. . . .
Caresses

The morning of December 9 was sunny and clear. I sent my younger children off to school in the usual manner. They knew nothing of my surgery.

My husband planned to tell them when they returned home from school that I was fine, and after dinner they would all come to the hospital along with their grandmother for a nice visit with me.

The longer the delay, the more nervous I became. I could see our carefully honed plan going up in smoke. By now, the medication they had given me had caused my mouth to become drier than desert sand. And my back was killing me; lying for so long on a hard transport gurney in the little holding room outside the O.R. was taking its toll.

My husband, sensing the distress I was feeling, took my hand and, without a word, leaned over the gurney and gently rested his other hand on my head. I felt so homely with no makeup and that ridiculous blue paper hat covering my hair. However, I knew I was loved, and, as I looked into his face, a calm peacefulness came over me. How fortunate I was to have him for my husband.

My time finally came. Dan kissed me good-bye, and they wheeled me away with the usual comment about taking good care of me. I guess it wouldn't be very funny if those blue-clad people mumbled over their shoulders, "Take a good look, you may not see her for awhile!" The last thing I remember was the anesthesiologist trying to get his IV into my right wrist. He asked me if I was nervous and I tried to answer, but my mouth was so dry, I just nodded. He said I would have a slight taste of garlic in my mouth and no sooner said than . . . I was asleep. The next thing I was aware of was my doctor's voice calling my name and moving my face back and forth. She kept saying that she and Dan wanted me to know it was plan A. Plan A, I mumbled, plan A meant good news, and with that I began throwing up.

In the weeks that followed, I progressed very well. However, I would have days when I'd get frustrated to find out how weak I still was. I had lost my independence and was dependent on my family for my needs while recuperating. I feared something terrible would happen to them when I was least able to deal with it. I had always been healthy and didn't handle downtime well. But to put things in proper perspective, all I had to do was turn on the television. The Armenian earthquake victims tugged at my heart, and the triple train wreck in London was awful. Then, on December 21, we were all shocked and saddened when Pan Am flight 103 exploded and went down over the small Scottish town of Lockerbie. All 258 aboard and 12 more on the ground were killed in a terrible act of terrorism. Suddenly my life didn't seem so unmanageable.

. . . .
"Go for it, Mom!"

With the surgery behind me, and the holidays, too, it was time for more major decisions. January 1989 began my six weeks of radiation therapy.

My left arm was giving me lots of trouble. The lumpectomy was a cinch, but the axillary dissection wasn't that easy to recover from. The lymph nodes that were removed were disease-free—good news. However, I needed physical therapy to regain the movement of my left arm. My radiologist knew just the woman to help get me into shape for my six weeks of radiation. Carmella was not only a wonderful and compassionate woman, but, in my estimation, a real miracle worker. I couldn't help but feel how fortunate I was to have such excellent health-care providers.

Whether or not to have chemotherapy was the most difficult decision I remember making. I agonized over it. Nobody in her right mind would want to endure the side effects of chemotherapy if it wasn't necessary.

My patient and understanding radiologist helped me make this decision by posing a simple question that I pondered at great length. He said the odds were in my favor already for long-term survival, but there were no guarantees. Would I be the type of person who could put the question to rest and take my favorable odds? Or, as time passed, would I be second-guessing my decision not to take the chemo? If the cancer did recur, would I blame myself for passing it up?

I decided to take the chemotherapy, and something I'll always remember was my seven-year-old daughter's logic. As young as she was, she knew I was struggling with a hard decision. Since it was my arm that gave me the most trouble, we let the children think I had arm problems until the time was right to explain the bigger truth. The right time presented itself when my new 1989 diary arrived in the mail. My good friend and former college roommate sent me a new diary every year. Even though she and her family live in southern California, we have remained close.

Kimi, my seven year old, was excited to bring it to me so I could unwrap it and read the inscription Barbara always wrote to me. When I read it, I broke into tears. Barbara's message talked about the arrival of our middle-aged years, with the best yet to come! Oh, how I hoped I would have my best years yet to come. My daughter was, of course, puzzled by my emotional response to what was normally a lighter moment. I took this opportunity to explain what had really happened to me. She seemed to grasp the concept of taking medicine that would make you temporarily sick so that you could be well in the long run. She was able to visualize the chemo as little torpedoes tracking down the bad cells that might still be hiding in my body. After I answered her questions, she was quiet and content as I cuddled her. Minutes later, she went to her room and returned with something in her hand. I held out my hand, and she dropped a little red hair barrette into it and pressed my hand closed. She said it was her lucky barrette and it had helped her when she had to get her school shots before starting kindergarten. She wanted me to "be brave" and take the torpedoes, because she would take care of me when I didn't feel well. She wanted me to "go for it!"

What a joy she was. I wanted to live to see my daughter grow up, and I would do all in my power to have this happen. I would also educate her early about what she needs to do to protect herself from breast cancer. Because of my cancer, she now has a major risk factor of her own.

Choosing an oncologist to administer my treatment was a high priority. I wanted to continue the level of compatibility I had experienced with my surgeon and radiologist. It took two tries to find one I felt comfortable with and confident about. Halfway into my chemotherapy program, I found out why this doctor had such a high level of empathy and understanding with all his patients—his own wife was dying of cancer and succumbed to the disease a month after my treatment was completed.

I personally did very well with chemotherapy, and, although I was prepared for hair loss, it didn't happen. As a matter of fact, I was very fortunate in that I didn't experience anything I could not manage. I had my injections on Fridays so I would have the weekends to recuperate. About six hours after the injections, I would feel like a toxic-waste dump. Oily slime lying on the surface of stagnant water was the visual image I had of the inside of my body. But within thirty hours of the injection, I was fine.

You can come close to leading a normal routine, but somewhere along the six-month trail of treatment, the monkey on your back takes an emotional toll. I broke down, cried it out, accepted comfort from those I loved, evaluated the battle I was fighting, and continued the charge. All things considered, I experienced more agony trying to decide whether or not to do the chemo in the first place. In fairness to those who suffer terribly from chemotherapy's side effects, it's important to remember that there are different treatment schedules and drugs, depending on the extent and type of cancer. Some chemotherapy treatments are very aggressive.

. . . .
The members of the club

Radiation therapy was a six-week treatment, and I breezed through with minimal discomfort and side effects. I soon felt like a bona fide member of the blue-clad club known as patients. The sad part was knowing the tropical fish in the saltwater tank adorning the waiting area would outlive some of us. We were all ages and from all walks of life, bonded together by a killer disease. We were protective of one another and never spoke in negative terms, even when the quiet depths of someone's eyes didn't match the cheerful exterior smile.

It was here at the radiation clinic that I became very close to one of our club members. It's one thing to speak about cancer to your family members and friends and quite another to speak about cancer to your peers. With peers, you are free to share your deepest fears with people who understand but are not emotionally involved with you, whereas sharing them with your loved ones is only likely to increase their anxiety. My friend, twenty years my senior, was a fascinating person who had traveled the world as a colonel in the army. We both shared a love of the music from *The Phantom of the Opera* and a fondness for "The Far Side" cartoons. He would bring cartoons that always brightened my day. We shared many good laughs together, making our challenges more tolerable. This special person was a life enhancer for me, and I cherish the brief time I was able to spend with such a fine gentleman.

. . . .
Happiness will never be the same

As I approach another anniversary of my cancer diagnosis, I am grateful to be alive. The personal growth I have achieved by means of the cancer experience is varied. I am certainly more appreciative of my life and my family than ever before. However, happiness will never be the same. I now carry in my heart of hearts a reverence for life understood only by fellow cancer victims. In my private moments, I wonder if I truly am disease-free. Will my children be able to write an obituary stating I died of "causes incident to old age"? My challenge is dealing with my fears of cancer returning and not letting them keep me from enjoying my life right now.

Cancer is so tricky and unpredictable, yet we want to hear doctors pronounce us cured forevermore. I try to guard myself against cancer's cunning and sneaky complacency. I have only to think of Gilda Radner and Jill Ireland, who had declared themselves "cured." But this treacherous killer reared up again, and the final curtain fell upon these two women entirely too early. Everyone is quick to tell me how important a positive attitude is. I agree wholeheartedly, but I will continue to walk softly and carry a big stick!

In conclusion, the advice I have is to be adamant about taking charge of your life and your body. Make time for routine health care. If we fail to take care of ourselves, we won't be around to take care of our loved ones. Also, get the best medical advice possible, even if you have to leave your hometown to do so. Many towns and communities are too small for state-of-the-art health care and can't provide the skills, services, or equipment needed to detect and fight cancer. Likewise, women should not be afraid of offending their local doctor, who may be hesitant to admit he or she can't provide the skills or services needed. Women must not view their doctors as deities but as partners in their personal wellness program. Questioning doctors in a respectful manner is our duty. Knowing the pros and cons of every treatment choice is vital. Making informed choices by reading and gathering information along with a second or even a third opinion is essential. Expressing your deepest fears to the doctor of your choice and enlisting his or her partnership is your responsibility. My personal experience taught me that the majority of professionals in the health-care community truly care about the well-being of their patients.

Something else I learned from my cancer experience was not to put off pursuing dreams and desires until "someday." Someday is now. I always wanted to tap dance. It took cancer to get me to make the time for lessons.

There is one thing I would do differently. I wish I had asked to have my tumor saved and stored in some medical freezer for future reference. As scientists uncover new information about preventing recurrence, maybe my particular cancer cells could be of value to me. I'm reminded of my grandmother, who lived through some very lean and tough times. She would always say, "It's better to have it and not need it than to need it and not have it."

Politically speaking, I'm very proud to have been part of the 1992–93 Washington, D.C., crusades mounted by grassroots breast-cancer coalitions from all fifty states. Our goal of persuading legislators to designate more tax dollars for research benefiting breast cancer was accomplished. Keeping the momentum and staying the course are essential if we are to put the odds in our favor. What we don't know can kill us.

A Month in the Life

Sherry Drabner

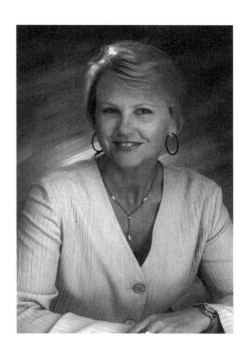

Sherry keeps a busy schedule as a mother with two children and as a model and account executive for a film and video production company. Sherry received training as a cosmetologist, and, as part of her job, she is a makeup artist and works with props and wardrobes. Her modeling career has developed a new twist since she developed breast cancer and now includes fashion shows for mastectomy patients. She enjoys waterskiing, racquetball, horseback riding, golf, and tennis.

Medical Bio

During the summer of 1989, Sherry discovered a lump in her right breast. The lump gradually enlarged over a period of nine months, and she consulted a surgeon who recommended a breast biopsy. The biopsy demonstrated a 2-centimeter infiltrating ductal cancer. There was also a palpable mass in her right lower armpit. She underwent a right modified radical mastectomy with immediate reconstruction. At that time, it was found that breast cancer had spread to five of twenty-four lymph nodes. Following recovery from her mastectomy and reconstruction, she underwent a course of chemotherapy, followed by a course of radiation therapy. Sherry then completed her breast reconstruction, including the reconstruction of a right nipple.

Shit happens.

The first time I saw that little quote, I had a quiet laugh. I laughed even harder when my boss gave me a large red pin with the same saying.

On March 1, 1990, I found out that some of the shit that happens isn't all that funny. That's the day they told me I had cancer. And let me tell you, things have never been the same. Change is the main thing that cancer brings with it, the main thing I've had in my life since that day.

At that time, I had two kids, was on my second marriage, and had finally developed a profession that would eventually make me financially independent and that gave me a great feeling of self-confidence. In January 1989, I had discovered a small lump on my right breast but didn't have the time or desire to have it checked out. My mother had had five operations for lumps, and they were all fibrous cysts. And during that year, both my father and my husband underwent surgery for possible cancer, and both had negative results. So I didn't feel the need to be concerned.

My lump was getting larger, but I still felt I did not have the time or desire to check on it. It amazes me now to think that cancer never entered my mind in respect to my lump. Late in 1989, my mother was in an accident and had major back surgery. The holidays were frantic and disappointing. I was very unhappy with my marriage, and we decided to see a lawyer. My lump was getting extremely large, and now I was concerned. I scheduled my appointment with the lawyer on a Monday and the mammogram on Tuesday. I really felt good about putting my life in some kind of order. Little did I know what was in store for me.

The rest of this chapter is from my diary, which starts at this point.

. . . .
Tuesday, February 27, 1990

Today I am finally going to have a mammogram. I have had a lump in my right breast for approximately one year. It is about the size of a Ping-Pong ball. I've known about it for so long that I kind of forgot about it until it became larger and protruded through the skin. Because I have breast implants, I thought they were involved somehow. I really feel there is nothing to be alarmed about.

The mammogram itself was a breeze, and the ladies there were very sweet and like family. Of course, the same question was asked over and over:

"Why did you wait so long to have it checked?" The only answer I could give was, "I didn't have the time." Since we had already established that there was a lump, we went further and had an ultrasound to see exactly how it was embedded. When the tests were completed, the attendant explained the urgency of having the lump removed for a biopsy. It was big and ugly.

. . . .

Wednesday, February 28, 1990

I had an appointment this morning with the plastic surgeon who performed my augmentation. He made clear the need to remove the lump as soon as possible, even though he thought the chances of cancer were only 6 percent. He scheduled the surgery for tomorrow morning at 10:30 A.M.

. . . .

Thursday, March 1, 1990

I really was put out by the fact that I had to go to the hospital and have this taken care of. I want this over and done with, and soon. I made it perfectly clear to the anesthesiologist that I have a tendency to be extremely ill after anesthesia, and we agreed to administer the treatment on a local basis. The doctor guaranteed I would remember nothing about the operation. Yeah, right!

They wheeled me into the O.R. and proceeded to hang a sheet in front of my face and scrub down. We finally entered the recovery room, and, boy, was I glad. The anesthesiologist asked about my recovery. I told him I was great and couldn't wait to tell him about the surgery. He told me to tell him all about it, so I did. I remember . . . I remember . . . I couldn't remember anything past the scrub down. He smiled, and we all laughed.

It seemed like forever before they took me back to my room. My mom and husband looked in the room and were obviously surprised to see me. I could hardly wait to tell them how great I felt and that the surgery was no sweat. As I was talking, I noticed that no one was looking at me. Mom was looking at Bob, Bob was looking at Mom. Mom finally looked me in the eyes and said, "Sherry Anne, the surgery did not go well. You have cancer!"

I couldn't believe what she said. I'm sure the drugs had something to do with it, but I was numb. The only thought that entered my mind as I stared into the hallway was my children, Kelly and John. How was I going to tell them their mother has cancer? What a devastating thought. My mother and Bob were crying hysterically, but I couldn't cry. I refused to cry. My mother reassured me that it was okay to cry and that I might even feel better. *No I won't. Just get me out of here.*

The hospital released me around 1:00 P.M., and I got to go home and wait for my appointment with the breast specialist in the evening. I had Bob call my friend Gloria and explain what was going on. He could hardly talk.

At the doctor's office this evening, I felt quite relaxed, but my mother and Bob were pretty strung out. When the doctor entered the waiting room, I knew he was the doctor for me. I could feel his compassion and concern. He explained what breast cancer was. The facts were astonishing, and I was amazed at how ignorant we all were about cancer. From the conversation he had had with the plastic surgeon, the doctor said he felt comfortable with a lumpectomy but would be more definite after he read the pathology reports.

He said I had a few weeks to think about the available options and that we would review them tomorrow. I was young and in good health, and these things were in my favor. I was not afraid. I was looking forward to tomorrow.

....

Friday, March 2, 1990

The doctor reviewed the mammogram, ultrasound, and pathology reports from the hospital. He examined the biopsied area of the breast and said he was not very happy with the location, but he would work with it. When he came to the other breast, he was suspicious of a cluster under my nipple, so he aspirated it immediately. THIS WAS A SURPRISE! He thought it was fine, but he wanted a second opinion.

Then he told me I no longer had weeks to consider the options. The cancer had invaded the lymph nodes in my armpit; he couldn't be sure how many were involved until we did surgery. It had proceeded into Stage 2, and he hoped that was as far as it had penetrated. He arranged for three tests: a bone scan, chest X-rays, and blood tests. These results would determine if it was too late to have a mastectomy. He said there was no sense in closing the barn door if the horse had already gotten out. I couldn't believe what I was hearing: I would have to wait—wait and wait—for the opportunity to have the right side of my chest removed. My God, what choices I have left myself.

....

Saturday and Sunday, March 3 and 4, 1990

These days seem to have lasted forever. I've told my story so many different times, I've lost track. So many people are concerned and shocked; they can't believe this could happen to someone so young and healthy. All I know is that I want the chance to have a mastectomy. I can't believe I'm saying this.

I found it most difficult to tell my children. To keep my cool and explain all the different procedures that were going to happen to me and what this meant to our future was not easy. I couldn't let Kelly and John see how scared I really am. They needed to know that I was going to do what had to be done and that in the end I was going to be just fine—maybe a little different, but just fine. My daughter took the news quite hard. She cried, and I cried with her. The knowledge that death could be around the corner is a lot to deal with, especially when you're fourteen and the death is your mother's. This was heavy duty. My son acted as if he didn't have time for this; I'm not sure he believed his mother could ever be that sick. I hope he will come around and understand what is happening and that I need his support and love.

. . . .
Monday, March 5, 1990

At the hospital for my tests, we drew three tubes of blood, and that went smoothly. My next stop was the X-ray department. There they injected me with radioactive dye. I was told to return in two hours and be sure to drink plenty of fluid, because this would ensure better results for the bone scan. Before I left that department, I had the chest X-rays. Now all I have to do is wait. Boy, am I getting good at waiting. No, I'm really not.

After returning to the hospital, I lay on a narrow table in my street clothes. The nurse tied my arms around my waist so they would not fall during the bone scan. You have to lie completely still while a machine starts at the top of your head and moves ever so slowly down to your feet. When it reaches your feet, it rolls under your body and works its way back up to the top of your head. While the machine was around my waist area, I could turn to the computer screen and watch the formation of my skeleton. It was awesome.

. . . .
Tuesday, March 6, 1990

Today I do not want to talk on the phone or be around anyone. I want to be alone. I don't want the doctor or anyone else to call to tell me any surprises.

I come home to find a message from the doctor's assistant. I don't want to talk to her now; it's too soon. It could only be more bad news.

I finally got the courage to call her back. She wanted to give me some good news on two of my tests. The results came back negative on my bone scan and chest X-rays. She will have the results of the blood work tomorrow when I go in for my exam. Wow, what a relief! It is looking good. I passed two of the three tests. Friday is slowly becoming a reality. Lucky me.

. . . .
Wednesday, March 7, 1990

It seems like an eternity since I talked to the doctor's office yesterday. I never realized how time could move so fast and yet so slow. I had lunch with some friends today, hoping the time would breeze by. It was great therapy.

The assistant had started my exam when the doctor charged in. Stuck to his finger was a Post-it note with a bunch of numbers—the results of my blood work. "Fine, fine, fine!" was all he could say. A sense of weightlessness came over me. I made it. I really made it. I told Bob to run out and call my mother, who had been sitting on pins and needles waiting for these results.

When the exam was over and all the gory details were discussed, I went to a friend's house for one of our scheduled group sleep-overs. This was an opportunity for all of us to let things resemble some form of normal. At first, we talked about everything but my upcoming surgery. But it didn't take long for the subject to get to my chest and what a good idea it would be to take photos—that way I could compare my old chest to my new one. I agreed, with the stipulation that my face was not to be seen. The night was great fun. The next afternoon, I felt anxious and decided to go home. I wanted some time to sort things out in my head.

. . . .
Thursday, March 8, 1990

My body is exhausted, and my eyes feel like the beach, all warm and sandy. These past few nights, it has been difficult to sleep, especially when I don't take those wonderful sleeping pills. I am definitely going to take one of those puppies tonight. I could really use the relaxation before my surgery. Bob and I didn't talk. We didn't know what to say except, "Here we go!"

. . . .
Friday, March 9, 1990

Here it is—the day we all hoped would come.

The doctor came in and played meat butcher with my chest. With his purple marker, he drew lines where he was to cut and a great big *X* where the mother tumor was located. Now I know how a cow feels.

The assistant talked to me while the anesthesiologist started to administer the drugs, and I started to breathe deeply. The oxygen mask came over my face and the last thing I remember was the assistant holding my hand and reassuring me that things would be just fine. The next thing I remember were voices calling my name. "Sherry, are you awake?" Without opening my eyes, I answered a very groggy yes.

The nurses said I could have a shot for pain. I didn't understand why I would be in pain until I moved. Oh, my God! It was incredible. It took my breath away. The nurse gave me morphine and that didn't even touch it. And now they wanted me to get up and go to the bathroom. Get real! What a major ordeal this was going to be. As I was assisted from the bed—looking more like a turtle on its back kicking for life—I began to feel nauseous and dizzy from the morphine. Then it came over me. I called to the nurse to bring anything that I could throw up into. Like lightning, she handed me the garbage can. Between the surgery, my period, and the vomiting, I felt extra special.

. . . .

Saturday, March 10, 1990

When morning arrived with my breakfast, I was eager to eat and enjoy a cup of coffee. Lunch was just as exciting. I'm surprised no one complained of oinking sounds.

Around 2:30 P.M. the doctor arrived. I was very anxious for him to explain the pain that was hindering my breathing and just about everything else. He unwrapped the bandage, and I gasped. The pain was blinding. He was amazed himself. It was apparent that the irrigation tube that ran from my rib cage up through my armpit to the top part of my arm was resting on the only nerve they have to cut for this process. RESTING? This tube was going out of its way to cause me severe discomfort. We all decided it would be best if I stayed one more night at the hospital, but I was taken off morphine. Lucky me! The next dosage would contain Demerol.

Now that my mind was somewhat clear of the surgery and drugs, the doctor explained how the surgery went. Because of my slender figure and good tissue, he believed the operation went extremely well. This also explained my severe pain from the drainage tube—there is no fat to cushion the amputated nerve from the tube. This is something I will have to contend with till it is removed on Tuesday. It's only Saturday now. Ooouch!

My husband walked in with a get-well card signed by his entire bowling league. This really touched me. I had no idea how I had touched so many people in so many different ways. My eyes filled with tears as I read all the special comments everyone wrote.

. . . .

Sunday, March 11, 1990

I woke up and hustled to clean up and eat breakfast. Home is where I wanted to go, but how was I going to function? The pain was incapacitating.

The doctor released me about noon. But the car ride home was quite an ordeal, and I really was made aware of how handicapped I had become.

My children came home from their dad's, and we visited until later in the evening. I suggested to Kelly that we bake cookies. I told her to mix them, since I was out of commission, then I would fix them on the cookie sheet. We were quite a team. It's amazing how the simplest tasks become major productions when you don't have the use of an arm. The pain was still unbearable even though I am taking pain pills every four hours.

I'm pooped, and it's time to go to bed. Bed—oh, no! I have a waterbed; there is no way I can get in and out of that. So it's off to the couch. This is going to be a long, long recovery.

. . . .
Monday, March 12, 1990

Kelly stayed home from school to play nurse. It was so pleasant to have her home to pamper me. She answered the phone and received my flower deliveries. The house looks like a funeral parlor. No kidding. I have never received this many flowers in my whole life. Cancer definitely has its perks.

. . . .
Tuesday, March 13, 1990

It's another one of those days I thought would never get here. Time to remove the drain tube.

The sensation of burning acid started from the tips of my fingers and rushed up through my armpit. I stared at the ceiling, expecting to see blood pepper it and everyone in the room. With each inch of removal, I thought I was going to pass out. I screamed rather loudly. In my many years of soft-ball injuries, tooth extractions, childbirth, and various accidents, I have never lived through such cataclysmic seconds of pain. I found it difficult to catch my breath; I was breathing so hard you would have thought I had run a marathon. I reassured the assistant that I was going to live, and slowly calmed down. Then a feeling of serenity and peace came over me. I could take a deep breath—there was no pain. The relief was beyond words.

The doctor's assistant fixed my dressing and proceeded to pump me up. She told me this would entail a small needle prick into the reservoir that led to the implant. After what I had just experienced, this was a piece of cake. She then asked me if I wanted to look at my new breast. I had to think for a second before I reached for the mirror.

I was pleasantly surprised and really impressed. I already had cleav-age—my chest was full. The scar was long and red, but it was not grotesque. Being slender proved to be to my advantage. I looked pretty terrific. I was very fortunate.

. . . .
Wednesday, March 14, 1990

It's so wonderful to be out of pain that I can't begin to describe the feel-ing. But today I didn't feel so well. By 2:00 P.M. I was feeling nauseous, then my worst nightmare came true—I started vomiting! Do you know how hard it is to sneeze, cough, laugh, or vomit with half your chest removed? By 6:30 P.M. I was out of control and called the doctor; at 8:00 P.M. he arrived. After I explained that Kelly had been sick two days earlier and John sick five days before that, he decided I had the flu!

I have to admit I was feeling pretty sorry for myself. With the surgery, an allergic reaction to the medication, the drain tube, and the flu, I was feeling lower than whale shit on the bottom of the ocean.

. . . .
Thursday, March 15, 1990

Today is sensational. It's amazing what one day can do. Physically, I am feeling much better. Mentally, I've been doing a lot of thinking. I'm nervous about my future and the events yet to come—cancer, chemo, my children, my personal relationship with Bob. It is all so confusing.

The past few days, I have been talking with another cancer victim. She had a double mastectomy followed by chemo and is about nine months out of chemo. I've enjoyed her outlook and very positive ideas regarding this disease. I hope to keep her perspective as time goes on.

. . . .
Friday, March 16, 1990

This is going to be the best day I've had since this whole ordeal began. The doctor called me first thing this morning and gave me the word: move it! He told me to shower, get dressed, go for a drive, and even pop in on work. Wow. I couldn't believe what he was saying; it was the best thing I could have heard. I can see how easy it would be to withdraw from reality a bit more as each day passes.

Bob came home around noon to assist me with my driving—or rather, my attempt to drive. I was not graceful or coordinated, but I got the job done. It's astounding how fast you manage when you have to. Off to lunch we went, where my boss, Paul, met us. It was my first time in public. Another obstacle tackled.

The rest of the day was quite busy. It was great to be out and about with the living. My physical disability is obvious, but I can manage. Attacking the difficulties is the best therapy I could ask for. Life is important and physical impairments are not.

. . . .
Saturday, March 17, 1990

I didn't plan many activities for today after my big jaunt yesterday. The biggest assignment was attending our Saturday-night bowling league. The members had been extremely interested in my progress. A majority of the league (sixty-four people) had already made some attempt to visit with me. Tonight everyone showed great affection. Comments ranged from how well I looked to the fact that they couldn't believe I was up and about. Of course, I didn't tell them how I had busted my buns to look terrific. After all, I did have an image to keep up, even if it took two hours to dig up that image. But I'm glad for every ounce of effort I put forth. It came back to me double.

A few hours into the evening, I noticed my chest was hurting and my arm felt like it weighed two hundred pounds. This was scary, because I really had done nothing to make my arm and chest hurt so bad. We cut the evening short.

....
Sunday, March 18, 1990

I'm taking it easy and anticipating a slow recovery from last night. Everyone is gone this morning, and I'm enjoying the quiet of the house. This afternoon, I plan to tackle the grocery store—this could prove to be interesting.

I'm not sure which was more challenging, putting the groceries in the cart or putting them away when I got home. After winning that battle, I wanted to cook chicken-noodle soup. Well, this was a larger undertaking than I had imagined. I couldn't even peel the skin off the chicken or cut the celery or onions. I couldn't lift the pot after it was full.

This is starting to piss me off. Bob and the kids have been spoiled for the past nine years, and this makes it more difficult for me as well as for them to cope with my helplessness. Asking my family to do something around the house is like talking to the walls. No one cares to go out of their way to help create a smoothly functioning home. It's only been nine days, and my house is in a state of delirium.

....
Monday, March 19, 1990

Today I had a haircut, and it has made an immense difference in my attitude. I decided to dress up and go out. I went to a restaurant, and the customers there were extremely friendly. When I got back home, the doctor's office called and requested that I come this afternoon instead of tomorrow.

The doctor filled the implant with 90 cc's of fluid. It feels so full and it's so high up on my chest that it must be under my collarbone. He assured me that if I wrap my chest in a bandage for a few weeks, my new breast will go where it is supposed to. Wow, what a relief.

....
Wednesday, March 21, 1990

What a long day today is going to be. Today I begin the chemotherapy orientation. I'm not sure what to think, mainly because I have decided not to even try to imagine what this is going to entail. My thoughts scare me to death (bad choice of words). The people who have had chemo talk very little about it. They just say that it was something personal and everyone does it her own way. Sounds exciting, huh?

Listening to the oncologist, I couldn't perceive how I was ever going to get through this experience. The actual operation was nothing compared to what's in store for me with chemotherapy. The doctor's game plan is for me to receive six months of chemotherapy—injections of two different drugs once a week and one drug orally each day. There are many side effects—hair loss, nausea, muscle cramps, sores in my mouth, fatigue, loss of appetite, and diarrhea. Lucky, lucky me. I can hardly wait. The doctor wants to start my therapy as soon as my breast implant is completely pumped up.

I'm feeling overwhelmed. They said there would be days like this when you can't talk or even write about cancer—this is one. I feel like I'm at Las Vegas, gambling and playing the odds; my destiny has so many variables, and I have very little control.

Tonight I was invited to be a part of a book project. Twenty breast-cancer patients and their families are going to write their stories. Each person's story will be a chapter in the book. I don't understand why I was there—I'm just starting. Most, if not all, were in remission with a few cancer-free years behind them. I can hardly wait to be in that category. There were many courageous and intelligent women I met tonight—apparently cancer shows no favoritism. Each story that was briefly told somehow managed to touch me personally. After the meeting, many of the ladies approached me and showed their concern. I feel like I'm in a special, elite club. I'm really not alone.

. . . .

Thursday, March 22, 1990

Today I am able to talk about chemo and how I perceive my future. The doctor shocked me with the statistics regarding my case. Having five of my twenty-two lymph nodes come up positive put me in a higher risk category. The facts are vague to me, but what I do understand isn't all that encouraging. All the tests I had before my surgery led me to believe that I was in the clear. What a false sense of security. To the best of their knowledge, the doctors removed all the cancer they could see. We just don't know if the mother tumor had any seedlings that detached themselves and are hanging out in my body. Without a substantial growth attached to an organ or present on my bones or lungs, there is no way to detect metastasized cancer.

I decided to get together with two friends to come up with a game plan to prepare all of us for what's in store for me. We read, talked, laughed, and even cried a little—but only a little. I will not waste the time and energy it takes to cry. There is nothing to cry about. I am very lucky to continue with my life. I told the girls about my apprehensions, and that helped. Their response was, "We'll be here when you need us." And I know they meant it.

. . . .
Friday, March 23, 1990

I find myself feeling irresponsible. I don't want to go to work, so I don't. I don't want to deal with people and tell everyone I'm fine when I'm really not.

. . . .
Saturday, March 24, 1990

I have three more days to think about chemotherapy. I try to keep busy and not give my mind the opportunity to wander.

I'm taking John with me to buy in-line skates. As soon as my arm heals, look out. It may not sound important, but it is. I'm at a stage in my life when I don't want to just talk about doing things, I want to do them. Today is another milestone in how I perceive my future.

. . . .
Tuesday, March 27, 1990

Well, folks, this is the day we've been waiting for: Chemo Day. Off to the hospital I go for my blood work. This is part of the procedure before chemo is administered.

After the blood work, the doctor invited me into his office and asked if I had any questions. All I could say was, "Let's get the show on the road." I weighed in and prepared my arm for the injections. The needle nurse then approached me for the kill. She was disappointed when she couldn't find a good vein in the left arm, the only choice available for chemo. She had to move down to the top of my hand. The needle had an extremely fine point and didn't hurt much. There was a very gentle touch and she slowly released the chemicals into my veins. I found myself thinking of anything but what was happening to me. She was able to change syringes without having to inject me again. Finally it was over. I made it.

The evening was really comical. Everyone called and wanted to know how I was feeling and what progress I had made. I felt like a pot ready to boil, except everyone was watching and nothing was happening. It was about as exciting as watching paint dry. My family was waiting for an ear or a fingernail to fall off; maybe with a fling of my head my hair would fall out. Everyone was nervous, including me.

After dinner I took my oral medication. Feeling okay, I decided we would all go visit my mother for her birthday. She was tickled to see me. I did find myself feeling a little under the weather as the night progressed. It took about three to four hours for that pill to kick in, just in time to go home and go to bed.

. . . .
Wednesday, March 28, 1990

When morning arrived, I opened my eyes very carefully. I felt a little queasy, like I had with morning sickness.

I've been thinking about trying to get away for a day or two. I'm tired of talking on the phone and telling people the same old stories over and over again. I need to catch up on my writing and just relax. I think I will do that tomorrow.

. . . .
Thursday, March 29, 1990

I still feel a little out of sorts. I'm anxious not to feel like this. That's a laugh—I still have twenty-three more treatments to go.

I didn't start my adventure till late in the afternoon. I had no idea where I was going. I ended up at a lodging in a small town nearby. What a surprise. It is very peaceful and quiet. There is no TV, radio, or clock in the room. The silence is deafening. Since I haven't been sleeping well, this will give me a good chance to catch up on my writing. I have put off writing because the thoughts of chemo would creep into my head, and I wasn't ready to handle them. Now that I have experienced my first treatment, I feel a little more at ease.

I walked the grounds and took my dinner to my room. Later I sat in the great room and just watched and listened for a few hours. It was so peaceful.

I am going back to my room to write until I fall asleep. I feel like the authors in the movies. It is appealing.

. . . .
Friday, March 30, 1990

Well, I didn't sleep any better with all that quiet. I found myself writing until three o'clock in the morning. I'm still feeling a little queasy but not real sick. I bet staying up late doesn't help. I went down to the hot tub this morning. It is strange to be in a swimsuit with my semideformed chest. It is beautiful and serene in the mountains. I will definitely come back here again. This is just what the doctor ordered.

. . . .
Nine weeks later

My story is still developing. I am nine weeks into chemotherapy and doing great. We are having a few problems with the veins on my only good arm. Each week we have to wrap my arm in hot towels and seal it with plastic. I wait fifteen to twenty minutes until it's soup, and then we take a poke. So far we have been fairly successful. There have been a couple of scary moments—including the time we blew a vein on the top of my hand and bruised my arm with the next injection—but we did it.

The doctor would like me to consider a catheter in my arm for easy accessibility for blood work and the injection of the drugs, but I refuse to have this done. I would have to wear the apparatus for the full six months and contend with it on a daily basis. At this point, the only time I think of chemo is the day I have the injections, and that's the way I want to keep it.

Three weeks after I started chemo, I had a throat infection that meant being on penicillin and a week free of injections. Other than that episode, I have it whipped.

The people in my life have been wonderful and very supportive. My mom and dad have had an extremely hard time, since this is not our first medical crisis. My brother calls me on a regular basis now. I enjoy the relationship that is developing, and I see it getting better all the time.

My children are doing well and appear to be adjusting to our new way of approaching the word *cancer*. We all have a sense of humor regarding it. A few weeks after my surgery, John yelled something to me, and Kelly interjected, "Gee, John, Mom has cancer; she's not hard of hearing!"

My relationship with my girlfriends has changed, and, for the most part, it has been for the best. Two have grown much closer, while one has dropped completely out of my life. It is probably the only negative in this whole mess. Her mother died from breast cancer, and my cancer brought back terrible memories and feelings that she apparently couldn't handle.

My relationship with Bob is not very positive. He has committed himself to helping me get through chemo and back on my feet again. When chemo is over, we will tackle the emotional aspect of our relationship and decide what will be best at that time. Meanwhile, we just live day to day. I might not be in love with this man, but I do love the man he is. I'd like to think we will both be better people when the dust settles, even if we no longer share the same life.

Having cancer has made quite a difference in my perspective. Having this happen to me made me aware of myself and my well-being. I never considered myself important—what a mistake that was. I am the most important person, and when I take care of myself, everyone will follow suit.

....
Two years later

I had six months of chemo; I went every Monday morning while I continued to work. Several weeks into chemo, my veins broke down, and a portacath was installed in the lower portion of my neck. That was devastating to me, but I have to admit it made the injections easier. I finished chemo weighing twelve pounds more than when I started and with all my hair. My theory is that we can achieve great results when we apply mind over matter.

I did six weeks of radiation, five days a week, without interruption. I used aloe vera every day and minimized the burn. I wasn't as successful with the fatigue. After five weeks, it hit me like a train, along with a highly irritating itch. But I passed with flying colors and still had a great result with my reconstruction and my implant. Once again, I had decided to do my time with style, and I did.

All I wanted for Christmas was a nipple. Five weeks after radiation therapy, I had my nipple constructed from a skin graft and finished the long and seemingly endless journey. My one and only goal was to finish all my therapies and surgeries by the end of the year. And I did it! I started 1991 with a clean bill of health and ready for the best years of my life.

I don't want anyone to think that this experience was a picnic, because it was one of the hardest things I have ever had to do in my life. But I did it. I did so well that people find it hard to believe that cancer happened to me. I have chosen to set an example of how life goes on and on if we maintain a positive attitude. I have had many wonderful people come into my life, and I have lost two darling friends to this ugly disease. One, Cindy Friend, was my age and left behind two lovely teenagers. I would like to acknowledge Cindy and the courage she gave to me to keep fighting. She opened many doors, and I will never forget her.

My life is always busy but not too busy for the things that are important—especially ME. I am very aware of life and try to live it every day, whether I'm happy or sad. I'm lucky to be here and experience the ups and downs and learn from them. There was a time, six months after all the dust settled, when I felt I had to have things happen immediately, if not sooner. It was difficult at first, but with some professional help, I was able to get a grip on life and put it in proper perspective.

I have continued my modeling career, including appearances in fashion shows for victims of cancer, and have helped many women who have had to consider reconstruction after surgery. I'd like to think that I have touched their lives and made their choices easier.

Restoring Perspective

Stephanie Zimmer (nurse-practitioner)

When I was asked to write a chapter for this important book, I began to reflect on the various experiences of which I had been a part and realized how much each individual had affected me and the influence my work with them had had on my life.

In theory, it seems that a health-care provider would be able to remain distant from the emotional aspects of dealing with breast cancer. After all, I am there to do some preoperative teaching, assist in surgery, and provide post-operative care such as removing stitches and changing dressings. Easy enough, right?

Guess again. Although I have not had the experience of coping with breast cancer personally, I am anything but distant from the experience.

There is probably nothing more important about this job than being able to convey some genuine warmth and caring to an emotionally distraught individual and taking the time to answer questions. That is when I begin to confront the real culprit—time. There are never enough hours in the day to meet everyone's expectations. That can be very frustrating. But knowing how therapeutic a hug or a quick phone call can be is very rewarding. Life is tough enough even when things go right—all of us could use a helping hand when they don't.

The real challenge I face is finding a balance between reward and burnout. It can be really tough to recall the many thankful patients you have had when you have a patient grilling you over the phone because she or he was only able to comprehend about 20 percent of the explanation you have already given twice. It can be very difficult to react in an appropriate manner and maintain composure. Sometimes I get so involved that I have to cry with the patient. Other times, I feel like screaming back and reminding the patient I did not give her this cancer. But I know that from the patient's perspective, the experience can be overwhelming. Treatment for breast cancer is a complex process of comprehending the treatment choices and making difficult decisions. Therefore, the stress levels go sky-high and the emotional baggage mounts.

Dealing with patients who are trying to cope with the fear of cancer has enabled me to witness the height and depth of human emotions, from sheer joy and complete relief to apprehensive anticipation and raw anger. It still amazes me to see the response a patient may have after receiving a diagnosis of breast cancer. I have seen all types of reactions, depending on the individual, her foundation of life experiences, and her support network.

The knowledge I have gained from my patients cannot be acquired from a textbook. This invaluable information can only be realized via a hands-on experience. Many of the patients have shared some very personal feelings, either intentionally or inadvertently, and this has forced me to examine my own fears of cancer and reevaluate my values and priorities in life.

I have come to realize that life really is short. It is impossible to pack in all the living we want to do; therefore, good health becomes more and more important. My gratefulness for this blessing has increased, not only for myself but for the patients to whom we have been able to restore it. I am learning to savor the moment and enjoy the little things in life that mean so much. Quality of life has become a very important issue to me. I guess that's what happens to us when life as we know it is threatened by an outside intruder over whom we have little control. In most cases, the die has been cast and we must all remember—patients and providers alike—that we cannot change what happens; the only thing we can change is how we react to that event in our lives.

Allowing each individual to respond in his or her own way, regardless of the ramifications of those decisions, has been a difficult aspect of this role. I feel it is the respectful thing to do. After all, patients are individuals who must realize their feelings are important. Many times I have borne the brunt of an angry patient lashing out, and it can be very difficult not to take those comments personally. But that is when I must remember that each patient must go through a process very similar to the grief process associated with death and dying. They must come to accept the diagnosis of breast cancer and get on with the business of living. But to reach that end point, they will many times go through periods of denial, anger, depression, and grief.

The challenge of this position is being able to identify where each person is on that spectrum of human emotions and intervene in the appropriate manner to enable that person to best cope with the decision at hand. It seems that the best way to approach this task is to take one step at a time and provide only the amount of information you think she can assimilate. If I can remember not to overwhelm the patient, she is much more likely to be accepting of the circumstances, and that usually favors a quicker recovery.

Becoming a co-facilitator for a support group for women with recurrent or metastatic breast cancer has reaffirmed my belief in the benefit of support groups. Women who have faced the same circumstances and experiences are given a chance to share the pain and the solutions. There are few resources available that are more comforting. I have seen firsthand the immense benefit that can be gleaned from such a small investment of time. A support group can help women realize that acceptance of their diagnosis is a process that takes time. And I hope I can always maintain a perspective that allows me to display compassionate and genuine care for those who are faced with this devastating disease process.

Finding Sources of Strength

How do we find ways to support ourselves in times of crises? For women faced with breast cancer, the answers are as varied as those posing the question. The authors in this section read widely, questioned themselves and others, turned to their churches and spiritual beliefs, examined their lifestyles, and became involved in support groups and political activism.

In "Questions and Answers," the author researched her disease thoroughly at the library and discovered that knowledge does mean power. The author of "How Long a Fuse?" learned through her search for information how important it is to have some control over her treatment and the direction of her life.

"One Hell of a Woman" tracks one woman's progress from crying on the day of her diagnosis to leading the campaign for a postal stamp commemorating women with breast cancer. And in "Today is the Day," the author shares her thoughts on the causes of breast cancer and what she has learned about living with the disease.

Questions and Answers

Joy Rogers

Teaching and being involved with young people offers great satisfaction to Joy. She has B.S. and M.A. degrees and has taught home economics for the past thirteen years, including the time during which she was undergoing the medical care related to her colon and breast cancers. During the summer, Joy works in teen camps and, lately, in "The Community

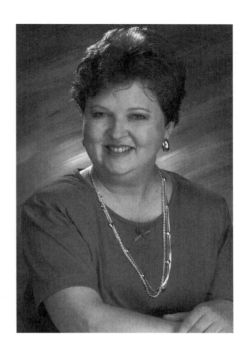

of Caring" program. Her other interests include book clubs, ballet, plays, dancing, and almost any vocal and some instrumental music. She sews wedding dresses and is engaged in scherenschitte *(German paper cutting). Outdoor activities include hiking, mountain biking, and somewhat spontaneous travel.*

Medical Bio

In February 1982, Joy was diagnosed as having a cancer of the rectum. This led to a partial colectomy and a permanent colostomy. She has had no recurrence of the rectal cancer, but in July 1984, she discovered a lump in her right breast. A subsequent biopsy proved that this was a 4-centimeter tumor. She underwent a right modified radical mastectomy with no findings of metastatic tumor in the lymph nodes. Following recovery from surgery, she underwent radiation to the chest wall. Six months after the mastectomy, she went through a breast reconstruction procedure.

During the following year, Joy underwent minor surgical revisions of her reconstruction. In July 1988, she developed a lump just beneath the skin but superficial to her reconstruction prosthesis. She also had a firm lump develop in the left breast. The left breast lump was found to be a benign tumor. However, the lump on the right side was a recurrent cancer. At that time, she underwent an extensive evaluation for the presence of other sites of potential breast-cancer recurrence, and none were found. Joy had a second course of radiation therapy and six months of chemotherapy.

Joy remained well until April 1990, at which time a lump appeared on her right chest wall. This was surgically excised and found to be another site of locally recurrent breast cancer. Again, she returned for localized radiation therapy to her right lateral chest wall and was placed on Tamoxifen. Joy was just beginning to recover from this treatment when she began experiencing pain in the right side of her upper abdomen. The evaluation of these symptoms revealed the presence of gallstones, and in October 1990, she underwent a cholecystectomy.

As a child, Joy had severe scoliosis. She underwent three major surgeries to fuse her spine and had extensive radiation exposure as a result of a very large number of X-rays. This exposed her intestinal tract and her chest wall to doses of radiation that are believed to have contributed to her breast cancer and colon cancer. At this time, Joy continues to take Tamoxifen and has no evidence of any recurrent colon or breast cancer.

Throughout my first twenty-eight years, I had several medical challenges, including scoliosis surgeries, back braces, and body casts. But I had overcome those problems and was enjoying my life and my career.

. . . .

How could this be happening to me again?

Then, in the winter of 1982, I was faced with my biggest challenge to date: the discovery of colon cancer. Part of my colon was subsequently removed. Two years later, on a checkup visit to my doctor, I planned to question him about some concerns I had. During the preceding month, I had felt an unusual fullness on one side of my breast, accompanied by a rust-colored discharge. But instead of voicing these concerns to my doctor, I just asked him what my chances were of getting cancer again. He told me my blood test (CEA) was lower than it had ever been. This was a good sign. Little did I know that this particular blood test was a colon-cancer check and not used for other cancer detections. He was so positive about my condition that I decided not to ask him any more questions. Besides, I didn't feel sick.

But the following month, I still had the discharge and also thought I could feel a lump. I was immersed in graduate work and didn't have time to be concerned about my health. Still, I worried constantly and couldn't concentrate, so I finally decided I had to do something about the lump. I made an appointment with a local health center.

As I left for the center, I felt foolish. I was afraid they would tell me that nothing was wrong and I was just imagining things. At the doctor's office, the nurse practitioner said she could not find anything. I was about ready to head for the door, gown and all; it was embarrassing to have imagined the worst. She called in the doctor to confirm the diagnosis; the physician could not feel the lump and showed no real concern but decided to order a mammogram. After some convincing, the hospital technician said the mammogram showed calcium deposits. I didn't know how important these deposits were.

I made a trip to the library, not for graduate studies this time, but for medical research on calcium deposits. It was not an easy task to wade through the medical books and journals, but finally I found a medical journal that stated that calcium deposits could be a sign of cancer, although this was not always the case. The next twenty-four hours brought a tremendous amount of anxiety. I remembered my previous experience with colon cancer and the devastating effect it had on my feelings of self-worth. I was still trying to accept the permanent use of a colostomy, the surgical consequence of colon cancer.

A flood of questions came to my mind: Did I now have cancer in my whole body? How could this be happening to me *again?* Did I do something to bring this on? Should I have had a different treatment last time? Would my breast be removed? How could anyone ever love me with such a disfigured body?

On my next visit to the medical center, I was referred to a surgeon. The calcium deposit looked suspicious, but the surgeon could not be sure until a biopsy was performed. If it were cancerous, he would remove my breast. I wanted to make that decision. I felt that he had no right to make it for me. It was my body. In the long run, I might have to have a mastectomy, but before I had it done, I wanted to check out another opinion.

After the biopsy, the surgeon informed me that the lump was cancerous. Because I didn't feel comfortable with him and was not convinced of his competence, I decided to change doctors. When I told him of my decision, he tried to put emotional pressure on me by telling me that he had cancelled his family vacation in order to perform the biopsy. He was also reluctant to relinquish my medical records. Looking back, changing physicians was one of the best decisions I made. I needed a physician to whom I could talk freely, one who would have enough patience and time to answer my many questions. It was important to me to feel comfortable with the proposed treatment plan.

My education on breast cancer began with my new physician. He patiently listened to me and answered all my questions. He set aside time to discuss my cancer in detail and presented all of my options through drawings and explanations of the X-rays; he explained that the options depended upon what was found during surgery. The days were crammed with months worth of learning. As a precautionary measure, a series of tests were scheduled before surgery to make sure the colon and breast cancer had not spread. My new physician's thoroughness built my trust and confidence in him.

When I told my family by telephone that I had cancer again, my mother became very quiet, offering only a few comments. Then she responded that she would be there when I had surgery. I asked her to tell my father, because I remembered how hard he took it when I told him I had colon cancer. He spent time trying to find another way to correct the problem without surgery. I was his daughter, and he didn't want me to hurt. More than anything, I had wanted him to approve of my decision, but he hadn't been able to do so at first.

I didn't realize how all of this had affected my mother until later. Just before surgery, she commented that if it was my time to go, then it was to be. I was so upset that I wanted to shake her to help her understand that I was going to be all right. I was determined I would beat this disease and make it.

Surgery revealed that the tumor was too large to save the breast. When the bandages were removed, there was only a flat wall with a scar. I could not contain the loss I felt. I cried until my head hurt. Every time I undressed, I faced this reminder of my loss. Reconstruction had been mentioned, but to me it didn't seem like an option: I had already had too many surgeries and dreaded each time I had to undergo anesthesia. Besides, reconstruction seemed like such a vain idea. I told myself I didn't plan to get married, so why should I go through it? The first time I went out in public, I put on a brassiere and began to cry as I stuffed one side with cotton. I was afraid of other people's reactions. Luckily, I had a friend who helped me through that first experience.

. . . .

Why me? Did I bring this upon myself?

Radiation therapy followed surgery. With mixed feelings, I arrived for my treatment. When I entered the radiation room, I was surprised to see five male university students. I felt like I was on exhibit as I pulled down my gown for the treatment. My privacy had been invaded without my permission. I left the hospital ready to explode. I felt desperate and despondent. Longing for someone to reassure me that I was still a human being whose privacy had meaning, I drove past a friend's house, hoping she would be home. Her car was not there. But as I entered my apartment, the phone rang. Somehow, she was prompted to call and answer her friend's silent plea.

With great difficulty, I told my radiologist I was not coming back. I was unable to give him an explanation because I felt too embarrassed and guilty. I felt I had done something wrong. When the doctor realized what had happened, one technician was assigned to me, and I returned for treatments. I was still emotionally on edge every time I went, but I completed the five weeks of treatment.

Physically, the treatment was not that difficult, but I found myself unprepared for the psychological impact. I was jealous of the other patients because I didn't have the support of a friend or husband with whom I could talk freely about my feelings. I vented my frustrations on the doctors, the same people who were trying to treat me. How I hungered for affection and concern from anyone who would listen and understand. One day a woman sitting with her husband introduced herself. She talked about how angry she was about her breast cancer and how she had cried many times. It was nice to know that I was not alone and that I was not crazy.

As I went through this experience, I asked myself, "Why me? Did I bring this upon myself?" Deep in my heart, I knew I had not, but I desired to find some reason for it. Hadn't I had enough? What was I to learn from this? What could I do to be happy again? Would people look at me and see only the disease, or could they see a person who needed love and acceptance? I didn't want others to know about my disease for fear it would alter how they responded to me. I wanted them to see the real me.

As I recovered from surgery and radiation, I struggled with my feelings of frustration. Without allowing myself the right to recover at my own pace, I compared myself to others and to their progress. I wanted to be as capable as anyone else. Eventually, I had to create a new, stronger inner being. By recognizing what I could do or what I had done well, I began to develop pride in myself.

. . . .

How would I feel when someone hugged me?

My doctor again brought up the subject of reconstruction several months later. I reiterated that I did not need it because I had no immediate plans for marriage. I did not realize that I needed the reconstruction as part of my inner healing. My mastectomy was a secret. Even when I really cared for someone, I was cold and aloof, afraid to trust and to be loved for fear my secret would be discovered. Because I had been rejected once, I was afraid other men I dated would reject me if they knew. I felt like a flower concealed in an ugly tin can. My doctor finally convinced me to undergo the reconstruction to improve my appearance and to give me the feeling of wholeness I needed. I had many questions about the surgery. Would reconstruction hinder any further discovery of cancer? Would they look natural? What would happen if the implants hardened? How would I feel when someone hugged me? What would the results look like twenty years from now? Did I have the courage to go through with it? Would I be considered vain?

Trying to find answers to my questions, I read as many current newspaper articles and books about reconstruction as I could find. After much research, I decided to go ahead with the surgery in February 1985, about seven months after my mastectomy. The thoughts of surgery scared me, but I wanted to feel whole again. I wanted to forget that I had ever had cancer. After calling the insurance company, I set the date and made arrangements for someone to stay with me the first few days after surgery.

The night before surgery, the phone rang—the insurance company had turned me down! They considered the surgery cosmetic rather than therapeutic. Didn't they understand that if I had not developed cancer I wouldn't even think about surgery? Without insurance, I would have to pay up front.

My physician assured me that this matter could be resolved. I continuously called and wrote the insurance company but with no results. Dressed in a business suit, armed with questions, and determined not to leave until I had a firm yes or no, I made a personal visit to the supervisor. I was told she was busy; I said I would wait. Finally, I met with the supervisor and refreshed her memory of the previous conversation. It had been over a month since I had been turned down, and I wanted some answers. I finally left with a letter of approval in my hand, and the surgery was rescheduled.

For the first three weeks after surgery, I couldn't reach, pull, or put my hands above my shoulders. I became creative and found out I could do a lot with my legs and feet, such as move boxes and furniture. I used a stick to knock things off the shelf when I couldn't reach them. I was unable to put them back, but that just made it easier to obtain them next time! Vacuuming was one less thing I had to worry about because it was on the list of don'ts.

As I recuperated, I began to feel whole again. My attitude changed, and my feelings about myself improved. I felt like me again. The reconstruction was not perfect, but neither is any human body. I didn't have to worry anymore if I was lopsided or if the padding would fall out. Because of the sense of freedom and satisfaction, I felt I had made the right decision.

During these months of medical challenges, I continued to work, taking just a few days off after the surgeries. In order to conserve energy, I eliminated graduate work and social activities. As I recovered, I questioned whether I should go on with my graduate studies. Family and friends thought that I was pressing my luck to even consider the hectic schedule.

I had almost decided that the obstacles were impossible to overcome when the wise counsel of a friend renewed my desire to try. I would never know if my physical health would sustain me unless I tried.

It was a rough summer, but determination and perseverance brought success within reach. I completed my master's degree, and more importantly, I proved to myself that I could not be defeated. In the fight against cancer you may not receive the recognition of a degree or medal for your hard work, but you can obtain a sense of pride for doing your best in overcoming a seemingly insurmountable obstacle.

....
Why hadn't she learned from my experience?

In the fall of 1986, my mother, who was then fifty-eight years old, told me that she had breast cancer. A year earlier, the physician in the small community where she lived had checked a lump on her breast. He was not too concerned but recommended that further tests be done at some time. The lump was not biopsied until later. Six months later, she found her breast becoming larger and firmer. By then, the cancer had already metastasized to her bones. A local cancer specialist told her she had about one year to live.

Again I questioned. Why couldn't I have this cancer instead of her? Because of my previous experience with cancer, it would have been easier for me to handle. I also didn't have to worry about children or a spouse. I wished she had told me about the lumps; I would have encouraged her to have them examined sooner. Why hadn't I gone home more often so she could have confided in me? Why hadn't she learned from my experience? I suddenly felt a great loss. She might not be around to see me get married or know of my future development and successes. She would not be here to see her own dreams for me fulfilled. Life didn't feel fair to me.

I was able to persuade my mother to seek another opinion. The second doctor suggested a different course of treatment, and she chose to follow it. It really bothered me that she was not more aggressive in checking out every detail of her illness. No amount of encouragement changed the way she addressed her illness. I wanted to take responsibility for my mother's behavior, but eventually I realized every person has his or her own way of dealing with a medical crisis. I wanted my father to be completely aware of her treatment, yet she would only share part of it with him. Several times after I questioned her about a procedure and its outcome, she would ask me not to tell him. It was as if she was trying to protect him from the pain. She didn't want him to worry when nothing could be done to change it. Several times this backfired. My father became very concerned when he found out that the cancer had spread.

I never thought that my mother's disease could be stopped permanently, but I always felt my own was curable. When I started taking the same drugs that had not proved effective in stopping my mother's cancer, I suddenly had a difficult time separating our diseases. If the drugs were not effective for her, how could they be effective for me? What was the success rate for this medication? Would my cancer follow the path of my mother's? How could I prevent this disease from ever recurring? What part did heredity play in these events? Was I doing anything to promote the disease? Whenever I felt the urge to compare our diseases, I had to remember that we were separate individuals with two distinct types of breast cancer and that our treatments and results would be different.

A year later, in 1987, my mother developed soreness in her hips and had trouble riding in a car. The cancer had spread. Her hips needed radiation, and her hormonal medications were changed. She later received chemotherapy. The hormonal drugs and chemotherapy gave her an extension of life, for which she was very grateful. Rather than have just one doctor treating her, she had specialists in the areas of surgery, radiation, and oncology who had access to updated medical knowledge. The choice to leave her own community for health care was difficult but made a difference in her survival. My mother would not have lived for over four years beyond the first diagnosis had it not been for the treatment plan and the optimism of her doctors, along with her own determination to survive and raise her sons.

. . . .
What are the side effects?

In the summer of 1988, I found a lump in the center of my right breast near the previous mastectomy scar. It was the size of a pea and very defined. When I asked one doctor if I should be concerned, he told me not to worry about it. Later I went for my yearly mammogram. I tried to find out the results before leaving on a vacation but was told to contact my surgeon for the results. Unable to reach him, I left for three weeks, wondering whether I had developed cancer again. I told myself I had two choices: I could worry about it the whole time I was gone, or I could live it up because I might have to face the recurrence of the disease when I got home. I chose the latter and had a wonderful time. These memories helped me through the grueling six months that followed.

Yes, I had cancer again. Two new lumps had appeared. A medical tumor board suggested that I have extensive radiation combined with chemotherapy. The thought of endless treatments made me very apprehensive. Again I questioned. How long would the treatment be? How often? What were the side effects? Would I lose my hair? How successful was the treatment? What were the benefits and risks? Would the drugs cause sterility? If I could get pregnant later, what effect would the drugs have on my future child? What would be the results if I decided not to undergo the chemotherapy? Would there be drug withdrawal? What would happen if I just couldn't take it and stopped in the middle of the treatment? Could I continue with work?

I still desired and dreamed of having a family. Would this make me infertile? The real question I needed to ask was: which was more important, life or the ability to create life? And yes, chemotherapy could make me infertile. Tearfully, I chose chemotherapy treatments and possible infertility, knowing that the treatment might prove to be ineffective in controlling my cancer.

I made a plan of action. Because there was the possibility of losing my hair, I looked for a place I could buy a wig. My hair became thin, but I didn't lose it. To accommodate the thinning, I just cut my hair shorter. On the days I received my shots, I would rent funny, lighthearted videos to distract myself and to help the rough days pass quickly. That worked fine for the first three weeks. On the fourth week, the electricity went out. For six hours, I called anybody who would talk to me about anything just so the time would pass.

In the following weeks, I returned to teaching and faced the ultimate challenge. I received my shots on Fridays because then I had the weekend to regain energy in order to make it back to work on Monday. On Mondays I planned less strenuous activities, saving those for Wednesday and Thursday. With the assistance of my principal, work partner, and other associates, I was able to function with dignity. I told myself I had to keep going because if I stopped I was afraid I would give up. As a result, I pushed myself to do everything I felt an obligation to do.

The medication, prednisone, gave me the delusion that I could do anything with endless energy—and then I would fall apart with exhaustion. Emotionally, I didn't feel I had control. All my physical problems seemed to escalate. Sores on the inside of my throat caused by radiation made it difficult to talk for the prolonged periods that were a necessary part of my work. I developed a dislike for many foods. I felt like a robot. Restless sleep at night added to my problems. I forced myself to function but continued to feel angry at the disease. I wondered if my attitude was faulty. My mother also came to stay with me during frequent checkups for her breast cancer. As the weeks wore on, I was torn between giving daily support to my family, fulfilling my work obligations (which often took evening time), meeting my home responsibilities, and preparing for almost weekly visits from my parents in a way that would not inconvenience my roommate.

After two months of chemotherapy, I couldn't go on. I felt useless and unsuccessful. Writing out the pros and cons of chemotherapy didn't help. The con list, reasons for not continuing with chemotherapy, seemed to grow. I didn't even know if the chemotherapy was killing the cancer cells. The positive effects of the chemotherapy weren't evident. Cancer might still recur. My life was unproductive, and I was unable to fully carry out my responsibilities at home and work. I was unhappy and tired of being tough. The only statement for the pro list was that chemotherapy *might* be killing unseen cancer cells and this in turn *might* prolong my life. Previous plans for making it through the rough times were not working. No matter what I did, everything seemed to get worse.

I told my oncologist that I was not going to have any more treatments because I couldn't handle the stress. I felt like an emotional time bomb. After evaluating my symptoms, he suggested that I see a psychiatrist. I agreed to go. I had had an occurrence of severe depression once before, when I had colon cancer. Once again, depression was coinciding with an illness. Antidepressants corrected the chemical imbalance caused by the extreme stress, and the depression ceased. I continued with the remaining four months of chemotherapy treatments.

As the weeks went on, my coping skills improved. Instead of an obstacle, work became a blessing with beneficial results. It gave me a sense of order in my otherwise deranged life. I discovered new ways of dealing with immediate problems. I used a tape recorder at school to present lessons that were repeated during the day. The students assisted with presentations and listened more closely so I didn't have to repeat instructions. Films or other means of instruction helped on difficult days. I tried to create good days when I could laugh and smile at the world; I read jokes and listened to motivational tapes. The day before my chemotherapy treatment, I rewarded myself by doing something fun or enjoying favorite foods. When I was feeling miserable, I would think of something new and exciting to do the following week. By simplifying home and work responsibilities, I was able to feel satisfied with my own efforts. Finally, I told myself it was okay for me to have a bad day, just as long as I didn't make a habit of it.

. . . .
Could you measure its effectiveness?

Near the end of my treatment, I asked my oncologist very seriously, "What major side effects will I feel when I finish chemotherapy?" He replied with a smile on his face, "You will feel better!" I had to chuckle. How true his statement was. With the completion of chemotherapy, I immediately began to feel a new surge of life, a greater appreciation for my existence. As my energy increased, I wanted to do so many things. It was as if I were seeing the world through eyes never used before. I was just happy to be alive.

During the summer of 1989, my implants were replaced because my muscle contracted. After surgery, I was concerned and wanted to know how to keep them from contracting again. I was fearful of the surgical process and didn't want to repeat it. Radiation often hinders and complicates the reconstruction process because the skin loses some of its elasticity. I was grateful that the new implants felt better and were more comfortable. I had a scheduled follow-up visit with my oncologist on Friday, April 13, 1990. Remarkably, the night before, when I was adjusting my brassiere under my arm near my shoulder blade, I felt a lump. It was not one of the usual areas I would cover in my self-exams. The lump did not disappear when I moved my arm. I lay in bed wondering if the cancer had recurred. I was so grateful to have a concerned oncologist who immediately said that it must be examined and removed.

Two malignant tumors were removed, but since they were in capsule formation, I did not need chemotherapy, only six more weeks of radiation treatment. It was startling to realize that the previous chemotherapy had not been effective in killing these tumors. My doctor recommended hormonal therapy. This brought with it another list of unanswered questions. Why was it not used before, instead of the chemotherapy? Would a more powerful chemotherapy drug be effective? Which hormonal therapy was best? If I was to use Tamoxifen, how much was known about it? How long had it been used? What were the benefits and risks of hormonal therapy? What was the length of treatment? What were the side effects? Could you measure its effectiveness?

Finally, I accepted the challenge to use the drug and live with the side effects. Still, it was difficult to accept the fact that I could take this drug and never be cured; that is, I would not be free of any potential recurrence of cancer. Until now, I had always had the confidence that my cancer would not recur. Hormonal therapy could only delay or suppress tumor formation. I had the choice of waiting for the next tumor to show up or taking drug therapy in the hope that it would suppress tumors for an undetermined period of time. After consulting with different medical personnel, I chose to go ahead with the drug therapy.

I am still a little apprehensive about the therapy, but, given time, hopefully, I'll be reassured. Who is to say that I won't be in the 40–to–60–percent success group?

. . . .

Knowledge vs. fear

As I evaluate the progress of my disease and my ability to come to terms with it and continue to have a happy life in spite of it, I realize that most of my learning and subsequent wisdom were focused around one theme: Knowledge vs. Fear.

At the initial diagnosis, I felt a loss of control. By asking questions, knowing the details of different treatment plans, and making the decision to choose a particular treatment plan, I gained control. The more information I acquired, the more power I had to make decisions and deal with the situation. The fear of the unknown was often more dreadful than the disease. Obtaining knowledge alleviated my fears. Not facing the fear only magnified it and made things more difficult. Unnecessary energy is wasted with worry; fear cannot be overcome until it is acknowledged.

. . . .
Spiritual guidance

I sought spiritual guidance each time I had to make a decision, in order to feel at peace and to have the strength and courage to make it through the rough days ahead. The blessings I have received through my illness have intensified my faith and reaffirmed my belief in a higher power.

Many times I laid awake in the middle of the night, crying because thoughts of cancer tormented my mind and body. I knew there was a Supreme Being who felt, loved, and understood the makings of my spirit and who could heal the confusion and feelings of anguish that overwhelmed my soul. Faith anchored and sustained me. Different individuals—doctors, friends, religious leaders, and family members—seemed to appear at the most needed times and places. They had the inspiration to direct and assist me in sculpturing the pieces of my life. Each time I was ill, I developed new and lasting friendships, and gained knowledge and understanding. I finally realized the length and course of my life was in someone else's hands. A peaceful feeling replaced confusion.

. . . .
Attitude

Sometimes, for short periods of time, life looked hopeless. I found that if I endured the pains of loss, heartache, disappointment, or physical torture, they passed or lessened, and my ability to deal with them improved. When some people said that I would be unable to do something, I wanted to show them that I could lead an active, normal life. I wanted to make a difference— a difference in other people's lives. At the end of my life, I want to look back and say that I have no regrets and that I used my challenges to make my life worthwhile.

People said I had a good attitude, but what other attitude was there to have? Could I give up and commit emotional suicide? I could not control the circumstances; I could only control how I responded to my circumstances. I had two choices: I could die with cancer, or I could live with it. "Terminal" may mean "final," but everyone is mortal. Anyone's life can be terminated at short notice or no notice at all.

To help myself accept this, I surrounded myself with people who believed in me, I kept mentally and physically active, I listened to motivational tapes and read books about others who had overcome obstacles or challenges, and I participated as much as possible in outside activities that I enjoyed. But I also recognized my own limitations, and I learned to say no without feeling guilty.

The question I asked myself when I was irritated by unfinished business or the peculiarities of other people was, "Will this make a difference tomorrow or even a month or year from now?" What did it matter? Was it really that important? I saved my energy for the important matters of life.

. . . .
Dating

Several men no longer considered me a dating partner after finding out I had cancer. They lacked understanding and human compassion. Tributes were wonderful, and admiration was great, but what I really wanted and needed was to be loved and accepted for who I was. At the same time, I had to love myself if I wanted others to accept and love me. I learned that my encounter with the disease did not determine whether I was lovable, nor did it decrease my worth; in fact, I developed greater character because of it.

. . . .
Positive aspects of my cancer

I may not have great book knowledge, wealth, or fame, but I do know what it is to savor life and to make it worthwhile. By facing cancer, I learned how to live better. Cancer may have invaded my body many times, but that did not make me worthless. It increased my ability to love and appreciate my family and friends. Some of my best friends are medical personnel who have given me support along the way. My appreciation for the wonders of life—the ability to function, to make someone's day, to have moments of pleasure, and to have days of just feeling good—have greater meaning for me. I don't postpone things. I am learning to focus. The experience of being able to help others who have had cancer has been an uplifting opportunity. It has increased my understanding, my patience, and my acceptance of others' needs.

The statistical odds may be against me, but I am not a statistic. I am living proof that I have beaten cancer so far and will continue to do so! Fighting the battles gives me the courage and experience to go forward. I'm just beginning to sense my own power and courage. The discovery of my own uniqueness, of my own inner strength and loveliness, is just beginning.

How Long a Fuse?

Roberta James

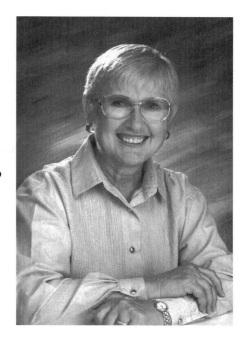

Roberta has a master's degree in English, with an emphasis in early American literature. She is interested in the history and literature of this era, and lectures extensively on the history of quilts in America. Roberta's lectures are accompanied by her quilt collection, which she has shared with audiences in several western states.

Roberta has served as a member of her city planning commission and as a member of the city council. She volunteers at a university library and at the breast-care center of a local hospital. She facilitated breast-cancer support groups. Roberta is a mother and homemaker with six children and thirteen grandchildren, and enjoys genealogy, gardening, camping, and sewing.

Medical Bio

Throughout her life, Roberta has enjoyed excellent general health. She went in for a routine screening mammogram at the age of fifty-one, which showed microcalcifications. It was recommended that she have a follow-up X-ray six months later. This demonstrated a change in the calcifications, which were in the upper portion of her right breast. In the interval, she had also developed an area of dimpling in the lower portion of the same breast. Subsequent biopsies demonstrated the presence of multiple sites of infiltrating ductal breast cancer in her right breast. She then underwent a right modified radical mastectomy; two of the twenty-nine lymph nodes removed at this surgery were found to contain metastatic breast cancer.

Roberta underwent a course of adjuvant chemotherapy and also had radiation therapy to her chest wall. Two years after her initial diagnosis and treatment, she underwent a delayed breast reconstruction and has remained on Tamoxifen. Her current health is excellent, and she shows no signs of any residual breast cancer.

Someone once said everyone has some kind of malignancy to battle. My cancer is a time bomb ticking away inside of me. I do not know how long the fuse is, or if the fuse is a dud and will not go off at all again. But then, all of us have a time bomb inside that will probably end our lives before we are ready. The difference is, my time bomb has a name: cancer. You may not yet be acquainted with yours.

Adversity introduces a woman to herself.

. . . .
I discover the time bomb

It was Saturday, July 2, and life was good. With four children married and only one left at home, I was looking forward to having the time to do some projects. I got up early to work in the garden, then came in to shower and cool off a little. Since I still felt sticky after showering, I stood in front of the mirror to fix my hair before getting dressed. As I raised my arm to comb my hair, I noticed my right breast was strangely indented. Anxiety was immediate. It was fueled by the thought that when I had my last mammogram in January, the radiologist had suggested a follow-up mammogram in about six months (or had he said four?) because it looked as if there might be some suspicious calcification, which sometimes predisposed cancer. I had not thought too much about it. Cancer was not a disease that ran in my family. I was healthy, happy, and had been busy with preparations for our son's wedding in May. The best of life was before me. I was planning a trip to New York and was going to leave on my fifty-second birthday to drive across the country with a friend.

It was a long weekend. I could not feel any significant lump in my breast, but it did not look normal. A mammogram was top priority for Tuesday morning. I had done breast self-examinations whenever I thought about it. I had had a mammogram five years before the one in January. I had been to cancer-screening clinics three times during that period of time, and I had

had an exam by a gynecologist the previous September. Surely I didn't have to worry.

Tuesday morning I had the mammogram at the small, friendly hospital where my son-in-law works as a radiation technician. He knew the personnel at the hospital and gave me an introduction to the radiologist. The radiologist invited me to view the X-ray as soon as it was developed. He told me that it sort of looked like there might be some suspicious spots in the upper outside quadrant of the right breast . . . and maybe I ought to have it looked at . . . and maybe if I were his wife . . . maybe I should have it done immediately . . . and who was my doctor . . . and maybe he should call and talk to him. So many maybe's and if's and so much beating around the bush. Couldn't he have been a little more direct? And besides, my concavity was on the lower outside quadrant of the breast, so why was he so concerned about the upper portion? I did not have a regular doctor, so the radiologist called a doctor, who suggested a biopsy. I could not imagine that anything was wrong with me. I had had no clue except what I had seen in the mirror, and I felt so healthy. The doctor set up the appointment with the surgeon for Thursday afternoon.

The surgeon, who I immediately sensed to be a very compassionate man, examined me, explained the options for treatment of malignancies, quoted survival statistics for breast cancer, then stated he could not see anything in the X-ray or in the physical exam to cause too much concern. We set up a tentative schedule for Monday morning when, I was told, a radiologist would help locate the lump with a wire or needle. I felt very relieved. By Friday evening, I had not yet received confirmation of Monday's schedule, so I called the surgeon at his home. He confirmed the Monday morning biopsy and explained that after he had more carefully examined the mammogram and reconsidered his physical examination, he thought my husband and I should discuss which option to consider in the event of a malignancy, but that he would recommend a mastectomy at the same time as the biopsy.

All of a sudden, my odds were reversed. Instead of being one of the nine out of ten who would not have cancer, it looked like I could be the one who would.* I really only knew of one option, mastectomy. My mother's cousin had had a mastectomy many years ago and died at the age of eighty. I knew of only one other person who had had breast cancer, so I called her for feedback and support. She had had a double modified mastectomy and had been reconstructed two months later. She mentioned she was grateful that she still could use her arms. My goodness, was loss of arm movement a possible price for this condition? She was cheerful and positive and said that before she had had her surgery she had checked with her brother, an oncologist in Los

....
*The current (1996) statistic is that one in eight women will have breast cancer.

Angeles, for advice, and he agreed that mastectomy was the way to go if the lump was malignant. It was good to talk to someone who understood what I was going through.

I thought a malignant tumor was a time bomb that would explode any minute with fatal results. There was no time to lose. The sooner it was gone, the better. I was terrified, but, in the back of my mind, hope remained. I would wake up Monday morning and my world would be right side up again. Cancer wouldn't happen to me. Besides, if only one in ten got cancer, why should I worry?

Still, I was very much concerned. I went out in the yard to dig dandelions. Every one became a cancer I was surgically removing from the lawn. For every one I dug, there were several more, proliferating all over the lawn. I could not keep them under control.

I desperately needed comfort but was ashamed of my anxiety. Others had gone through this alone and had not asked for help. No one had held their hand. They were so strong. What was wrong with me? I wanted to draw strength from my church community, to have them share my fears so I could share their faith. At the same time, I'd think, no need to bother them; why get everyone upset for nothing? After all, I couldn't have cancer—no one in my family had cancer, and I was so young. Cancer only struck the old, didn't it? I could handle this little trial all by myself. Then that little voice deep down inside me said, "Do you think you are above asking for help? Do you think you do not need the faith and prayers of your friends? Do you think you can walk all alone, without support? Do not be too proud to call on God for help. Your pride can be your undoing."

I was scared and needed support, so I swallowed my pride, humbled myself, and asked for the faith and prayers of my congregation on the Sabbath day. Then I heard the spirit whisper to me, "It's okay, Roberta, it's okay."

"What's okay?" I questioned. "That I have cancer, that there's a good possibility I will die from this ugly disease?"

Again came the reassurance, "It's okay." The spirit gives us strength, not answers. A peace came to me then that had nothing to do with my state of health or my state of mind. It was a gift from God that comforted me and gave me strength in the weeks to come.

. . . .
We begin to defuse the bomb

As I came out of the anesthetic Monday afternoon, I hurt dreadfully. I did not need to be told that my worst fears were realized. Cancer. The word tasted black on my tongue, was covered with burrs, and I could not get it past my lips. I could not say the word.

The doctor told me that during the one-hour-and-fifty-four-minute surgery, he had removed my right breast, which had two malignant tumors, one in the lower outside quadrant and one under my arm. Only two of nineteen lymph nodes that were removed were positive. The doctor recommended calling a cancer specialist for further consultation and treatment.

The entire visit with the oncologist seemed to take about fifteen minutes and then he was gone, leaving me to contemplate my future and chemotherapy alone. I was later very surprised to read my medical history and learn that the oncologist had "thoroughly discussed" with me my illness and possible methods of treatment. The fee reflected this in-depth consultation, but my memory did not. I felt like I had been read my Miranda rights. I did not feel that I had any choices at all. And I didn't like the idea of chemotherapy.

How I handled the situation was more important than why I was afflicted. My husband had always said, "When life hands you a lemon, make lemonade." Where was that recipe for lemonade now? I only knew that somehow the experience of having cancer had to enrich my life in some way and bless the lives of those around me. I didn't know how, but making my experience with cancer work for me might be the only positive outcome I could find for the lemon that life had given me.

I had surgery on July 11. I started chemo on July 22. Facing chemo was worse than facing surgery. Before surgery, I still had a thread of hope that I would be spared a malignancy. Now I only hoped chemo would not be as bad as I expected and that it would do the job we hoped it would.

My husband went with me when I made my first visit to the cancer clinic. It was one of the most unfriendly places I have ever been (I'm not sure any cancer clinic could seem friendly when you're uptight and facing your first chemo). The women at the front desk were abrupt and cold, neither helpful nor sympathetic. They were almost curt when giving directions. Upstairs in the oncologist's office, the climate was no warmer. We waited a long time, watching old people shuffle in for chemo treatments. I wanted to run and hide. What had I done to deserve this? I felt too old too soon.

I was glad my husband was there to hear the statistics the doctor reviewed with us again, because he heard the odds for survival rather than for death. The doctor recommended a six-month regimen of chemotherapy with 5FU, methotrexate, Cytoxan, and prednisone, two weeks on and two weeks off. All I had to do, I thought, was survive for six more months.

I started chemo that afternoon, full of fear and reluctance and not yet fully recovered from surgery. The chemo nurse gave me an antinausea pill, explaining that some cancer patients didn't get nauseated from the drugs, and some didn't even lose their hair. I went home after a very long day, all stressed-out, and became nauseated.

The nausea did not continue after the first day, and I felt like I was making good recovery from surgery. I was tired, yes, but not incapacitated. I got up every day, did some light housework for a while, rested a while, did more tasks, and rested again.

I had been on chemo for about a month when my hair started to fall out. I was on the phone when I first noticed I was shedding; my hair was coming out by handfuls. What was worse than having my hair fall out was picking it up from the floor, the furniture, the pillow, the table. Everywhere I went, I left some of me behind. I bought a wig and hated it. I bought scarves and they didn't work. I finally found some pre-tied, cotton head scarves that had a place to attach a little hairpiece over the forehead. Although I didn't use additional hair, these worked quite well. Later, I discovered a small, supplementary hairpiece that gave fullness to the sparse hair I had left. I never did lose all my hair. Most of the time, I just combed it neatly. I was swollen from the prednisone and my self-image was at an all-time low. I was still glad to be alive. I looked forward to Christmas, a new year, and a return to normalcy.

When my hair did start to grow back (before the chemo was finished), it was terrible. All that new growth fuzzing over my scalp made the longer hair stand on end. I looked like I had stuck my finger in a light socket. That's when I really appreciated the hairpiece.

I finished my fourth course of chemo on a cruise ship in the Caribbean. My husband thought the rest and relaxation would be good for me. He had been very supportive of me during this period, and I knew he was struggling with accepting this illness just as I was. He had been at my side when I needed him, steadfast and secure. One morning as I was recuperating from surgery, I became impatient with him for some real or imagined slight. Then I realized my frustration was not with Tom, but with the whole idea of cancer, mastectomy, chemotherapy, illness, and mortality. But it was easier for me to be mad at Tom; I could handle that. I could not handle the cancer yet.

To wake up and suddenly find yourself on the far side of middle age is one thing; to explore that land of no return with a loved one who is also aging, to share the frustrations of a body that doesn't work quite like it used to, a body that says "whoa" and a spirit that still says "giddyap" can be a rich and rewarding experience. I realized how great a love and appreciation I have for this man who has been my husband for thirty-two years and still loves me in spite of surgeon's scalpel, chemo's debilitation, baldness, and encroaching old age.

A few days after returning from the Caribbean, I checked into the hospital with a low fever and lack of energy. I was hooked up to an IV and oxygen. The next morning, the oncologist's partner told me that the X-rays indicated I had pneumonia with scarring on my lungs. I would have only 35 percent use of my lungs for the rest of my life and would need to be on oxygen continually. That diagnosis really made me mad. No way was I going to accept the fact that I would have to be tethered to an oxygen bottle forever. My friend, a nurse with a specialty in stress management, encouraged me. I could develop the remaining 35 percent of my lungs to compensate for the loss. Don't worry, just relax, breathe deeply, and think positive. Lung experts were called in, more tests given, IVs and oxygen replenished, and ten days passed. Reevaluation indicated the inflammation of my lungs was probably caused by the methotrexate or Cytoxan or both and was reversible after all. My lungs began to heal.

The doctor had said I was undernourished when I was admitted to the hospital. I didn't know how that could be. My appetite was excellent, probably because of the prednisone. The doctor ordered three or four milk shakes a day, a food supplement, and all the good, rich foods I could eat. I called for a milk shake at 6:00 A.M. so I could drink my quota before nightfall. What a way to start the day. I was already drinking two quarts of water every day. With the inactivity forced upon me by illness, I began to feel bloated and miserable. I felt if I survived the cancer, I would be ready for the cardiac clinic. I needed exercise.

Soon I was walking around the nurses' station without my oxygen tank and using the IV stand for support. First it was just for two or three minutes, but before I left the hospital I was walking for eight to ten minutes at a time. What an accomplishment. I was on the road to recovery. Within three weeks of my release from the hospital I was walking two miles in forty minutes.

With the release from the hospital came a reevaluation of my regimen. Cytoxan and methotrexate were out. The oncologist decided that since I had had two-thirds of one regimen (four of six courses), I needed one-third of another. The one he suggested was a combination of 5FU, melphalan, and Tamoxifen. I was on chemo for one week, then off for five. The good news was that this regimen almost gave me a chance to forget I was sick or on chemo; the bad news was that instead of being finished at Christmas, I would have chemo until the Fourth of July.

. . . .
Learning to live with the bomb

The diagnosis of cancer had sent me into some kind of shock or torpor. At the beginning of the treatment, I put myself completely in the hands of my physicians. Whatever they suggested I submitted to without question. Then one day my son-in-law brought me the book *Alternatives* by Rose Kushner. I realized I needed to know more about my illness. I began reading everything about cancer I could get my hands on. By October, I was reading Simonton's *Getting Well Again* and was very depressed, thinking I was not only personally responsible for getting the disease but also primarily responsible for my own cure. I did not want that responsibility, but I realized that the choice to live or die was mine. I thought of how nice it would be to die, to be free of worry and cares, to be reunited with my son and my mother. I was not afraid to die. I made a mental list of all the pros and cons of dying, and I listed several positive aspects. I could accept death.

On the other side of the ledger, I tallied all the reasons I should live—a loving and caring husband, five wonderful children (one still at home), and seven grandchildren, with more to come. And the sun was shining today. It was a gorgeous day, and the colors were vibrant: golden quakies, deep green pines, blue, blue skies. The world was so intensely beautiful it almost hurt.

I chose to live, but to do so I had to take an active part in my own recovery. I started by using the imaging technique suggested by Simonton. I visualized the chemo and my immune system as army tanks with laser guns battling my cancer cells, which were cowering under the bed. After the battle, the debris was swept away by a very powerful vacuum system. The imagery was strong, and I worked on it systematically. After one particularly intense battle that seemed to last all night, I awoke feeling free of cancer.

I continued to read all I could find about breast cancer. I empathized with Jill Ireland's *Life Wish* experiences, found hope in Norman Cousins' *Anatomy of an Illness* and Bernie Siegel's *Love, Medicine, and Miracles*. I was awed by the immune system as described in *The Healer Within* by Steven Locke and Douglas Collegan. I was discouraged to think I might fit the profile of the cancer personality as described by Simonton, until I read Claire R. Farrer's battle cry, "Stop blaming the victim." She said, "I've done all the right things and none of the wrong ones and still had cancer. And I do not appreciate anyone, whether a lay person or one with initials after the name, telling me if only I'd done X or Y, or eaten this instead of that, I'd not have had cancer." I agreed completely.

I found through my reading that there is still much we don't know about cancer. It is a capricious disease, striking suddenly, hiding only to reappear in another organ of the body or never appearing again. But I needed now to be involved in my own recovery. When I changed regimens I asked my oncologist if he had any written information I could study about the new drugs he recommended. "There is an article," he said, "but it's full of scientific medical information. You probably wouldn't understand it." Then he added condescendingly, "But if you really want a copy, I'll get it for you."

I had a difficult time developing a rapport with my oncologist although I had great respect for his skill in chemically treating my cancer. He was basically a kind and gentle man but very cautious and reserved with his patients. I felt like a disease, a number on a chart, not a person. When he walked through his waiting room, he would not make eye contact with nor greet his patients. His distant attitude was reflected by the receptionists. I told myself that a cancer doctor couldn't get too close to his patients and keep his sanity. Still, I wanted to be noticed as a person. I wanted to be Roberta who has cancer, not a cancer patient named Roberta.

In talking with other women who had breast cancer, I noted how important they felt it was to have some control over their illness, their recovery, and the direction of their lives. Those women who were bitter and angry were often the ones whose doctors had not given them enough information for them to feel they had any control over their situation. Maybe this kind of anger, which demands answers to hard questions, is the kind that promotes survival. This feeling of control over some area of our lives is what Victor Frankl identified in *Man's Search for Meaning* as the secret to survival in the Nazi concentration camps of World War II. Those who ceased to hope, who ceased to feel that they still had control of their attitude, gave up and died.

I knew I could enhance my treatment by improving my diet, exercise, and attitude; these were my areas of control. A diet low in fat and cholesterol, rich in fruits and vegetables, and high in fiber could not hurt and would possibly inhibit, or at least deter, a recurrence of cancer as well as heart disease, arthritis, diabetes, and osteoporosis.

Daily exercise became a must. Although I had never before been willing to give up an hour a day for consistent exercise, now my life depended on it. I joined a group of neighbor women who walked three miles a day, five days a week. The group was compatible, and I soon found as much strength and support in the conversation as I did in the therapy of walking.

Attitude was the fun area to work with. I read that those with good attitudes were more likely to survive cancer, but what was a good attitude? And if good attitude was so important in the treatment of cancer, why did people with good attitudes get cancer in the first place?

I discovered that one of the cornerstones of a positive attitude was gratitude. I learned that my own life was happier if I looked for the worthwhile in life and actively expressed my gratitude. It was so good to see the sun shine in the morning. I was alive another day.

I drew a deep breath—I could use 100 percent of my lungs and I was grateful. I knew what it had been like to not be able to breathe deeply.

I was grateful for friends who stopped by for visits and for the gifts of food they brought, the words of encouragement and expressions of love. My son-in-law said the greatest difference he had seen in me since cancer was that now I had time for family and friends and relationships. I was rethinking my priorities, and family and friends were becoming more important.

I was grateful that I could do what had to be done each day. I would set goals for myself—cleaning the kitchen counter, scrubbing the bathroom sink, or folding the laundry. Everything else could wait until tomorrow. Then at night I would think of how much I had done, not how much wasn't done. I found I was really accomplishing quite a bit.

I also learned about submission. I was ill, and my illness and subsequent treatment put limitations on my activities. I explored those limitations, defined the perimeters imposed on me by my health, and determined to live as fully and completely as possible within those perimeters. I did not need to retreat into a world of hypochondria or self-pity. I redefined my life goals and set priorities. My life became fuller and richer because I focused on what was really important to me. I was submitting to cancer with strength and power.

I don't think I could have survived my mastectomy and year of cancer treatment as well as I did without humor. Surgery was not yet six weeks behind me when my sister and I stopped at an antique shop. On one shelf was a yellow pottery jug bravely displaying an 1874 ad for inflatable bosom pads, a dollar a pair. I couldn't believe the timing or the good fortune in discovering such a treasure. I still chuckle when I see it.

Maybe laughter does not enhance the therapy or cure the disease, but it certainly makes life more enjoyable. Any day that provides its share of smiles is superior to a day of rain. And illness spawns its own brand of humor. Being able to laugh at situations by not taking yourself too seriously disarms many a hurtful situation and puts others at ease.

I was on chemo for a year and radiation therapy for six weeks. I struggled through the posttreatment depression, and now, two-and-a-half years after diagnosis, I consider myself a recovered cancer patient. I like that term. Each day is a very special gift.

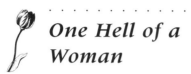

One Hell of a Woman

Betty R. Pittman

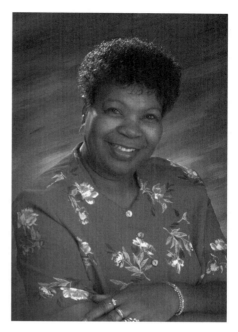

Betty is fifty-two years old, the youngest of six children. She is the mother of two girls and the grandmother of two girls and a boy. Betty works at a children's hospital and, in her spare time, enjoys golfing and reading. She is dedicated to her church and to finding a cure for breast cancer.

Medical Bio

Betty R. Pittman was a postmenopausal female with biopsy-proven infiltrating ductal carcinoma in the right breast. Betty first noticed a lump in her right breast while showering. She pursued the finding with a doctor and a mammogram. This revealed a suspicious irregular lesion in the right breast. No metastatic tumor was found in twenty lymph nodes dissected. Betty had a right modified radical mastectomy. She is currently well with no evidence of recurrent breast cancer.

. . . .
My emotions

I'm going to write this down so I can rid my brain of it and get on to the important elements in my life. Yes, I had terror in my heart. Yes, I wondered if I was going to die and not see my grandchildren grow up. Even now, that fear is still there, but I am learning to live, live harder, and live more. I had to abandon altogether the search for security and reach out to the risk of living with both arms embracing the world like a lover, to accept pain as a condition of existence, to opt always for total acceptance of every consequence of living and dying. This is about me, Betty R. Pittman, and life after the big C.

I was diagnosed with breast cancer on October 6, 1990. I cried for about an hour with a friend who had come with me to the doctor's; then I went home and called the doctor's office and talked with his nurse. We talked about what I felt and how I planned to deal with this disease, including whether to have the lump removed or have a radical mastectomy. My choice was to have the mastectomy with reconstruction. I was filled with a lot of emotion about my personal appearance and my insecurities. I tried to imagine what I would look like after surgery. I began crying again.

Later, I met Lucille Leonard, who was also a Big C survivor. She became my best friend or, as we say, my bosom buddy. Talking with Lucille assured me that my world hadn't come to an end.

. . . .

An abbreviated diary

O c t o b e r   1 0 ,   1 9 9 0 At 7:45 A.M. I am being prepped for surgery and crying the entire time. The surgery went well, and my doctor is wonderful, telling me everything about my surgery and my recovery.

N o v e m b e r   9 ,   1 9 9 0 I woke up at 5:30 A.M. with pain and swelling in my breast. The doctor's nurse advised me to come to the office. Fortunately, it was nothing more serious than inflammation of the nerve endings.

D e c e m b e r   2 0 ,   1 9 9 0 I am back in the doctor's office because my body rejected my implant and it is necessary to have it removed. I feel better as time goes by. I have come to accept this new disease with support from my family and friends.

F e b r u a r y   1 3 ,   1 9 9 1 The doctor discussed with me the idea of having another implant. But I am not sure at this point if I should have another one.

M a r c h   3 ,   1 9 9 1 I went to a boutique and purchased a silicone breast prosthesis. I liked the way it looked and felt.

J u l y   2 3 ,   1 9 9 1 I met with Vice President Dan Quayle at the dedication of our city's breast-care center. It was so nice to talk with the Vice President. He spoke of his wife, Marilyn, whose mother had died one year earlier of breast cancer. And there was a very delightful reception at the governor's mansion with some survivors of breast cancer.

December 9, 1991 I returned to the hospital for reconstructive surgery of the implant, and the surgery went well. By February I was having no problems, looking good, and feeling good. The doctor told me everything was going well and I could start seeing him every six months.

November 6, 1993 The doctor says everything is continuing to go well for me. Now I do not have to go to the doctor for one whole year! Yes! Yes!

November 8, 1993 A poem for myself:
May life always bring me the things most worthwhile.
God, give me the courage to greet each new day with a smile,
a purpose to work for,
a challenge to meet real satisfaction
to make my life complete always.
As I said, if I survive this disease,
I will be one hell of a woman.

January 6, 1994 A friend had asked me to chair a fund-raiser for a one-woman, one-act play called *Sister Girl.* I agreed to do this, with her help. It kept me very busy, but it was great. The play opened, and it was very successful.

April 29, 1995 I am off to Washington, D.C., with the National Breast Cancer Coalition, of which I am a member. It was a wonderful experience to see all of these breast-cancer survivors together in one place—beautiful women we are. We were all greeting each other as if we had known each other all of our lives. In a sense, it is an awful and sad way to meet friends, but you feel so good being with other people who have experienced the same trauma and feelings you have known. They become like a family with a common bond. It was the best experience of my life. We are taking these senators by storm, and I love it!

. . . .
Breast Cancer Awareness Stamp

Little did I know that Elvis Presley would be an inspiration to me. Because of the attention given to his commemorative stamp, I started to inquire about a commemorative stamp for breast-cancer awareness. I contacted the local post office and was told how to go about it. I began collecting signatures on a petition that read: "We, the undersigned, urge the United States Postal Service to create and issue a stamp commemorating the 2.6 million courageous women currently living with breast cancer in the United States alone." I shared this idea with other breast-cancer survivors, and they thought it was great.

I then learned that a breast-cancer survivor and postal worker in New York was also collecting signatures in a big way and writing to the Postmaster

General, and I was very excited to think that the stamp was really going to happen.

I submitted two thousand signatures, along with a sketch drawn by my good friend Martha Kelly of a woman looking over her right shoulder, a pink ribbon attached to the sketch. That sketch is now depicted on the official Breast Cancer Awareness Stamp, issued in June 1996. It happened!

Breast cancer is an epidemic that affects 2.6 million women and our families and friends. Eleven thousand of my sisters in my state alone have breast cancer. Although I'm very sorry that it has touched so many lives, it is exciting to be part of a campaign to increase public awareness of this disease. In addition to buying stamps, please continue to help fight breast cancer by doing monthly breast self-exams and having a clinical breast exam annually and a mammogram according to the American Cancer Society guidelines.

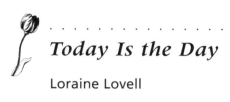

Today Is the Day

Loraine Lovell

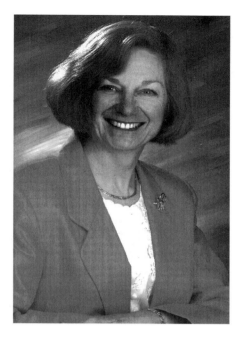

Loraine was born in Kent, England, and has been educated in such diverse countries as Australia and Jersey in the Channel Islands. She was a chief stewardess with British Airways in London, where she met her first husband before moving to the United States. After her divorce, she joined Eastern Airlines. Loraine is now a travel agent certified by the Australian Tourist Commission to promote travel to the land down under. She enjoys photography, birdwatching, gardening, and outdoor activities with her husband, Ray.

Medical Bio

On New Year's Eve 1991, just after her forty-eighth birthday, Loraine discovered a small lump in the outer right quadrant of her right breast. A needle aspiration was performed, and no malignant cells were identified. Because the cyst refilled with blood and fluid, her surgeon recommended an excisional biopsy. This showed a 12-millimeter intracystic papillary carcinoma with a 3-millimeter invasive component. Loraine elected to have conservation surgery with an axillary node dissection, followed by six weeks of radiation therapy. Her excised lymph nodes showed no signs of metastatic disease.

It was December 31, 1991. New Year's Eve. My husband and I had just celebrated the coming of the new year and had gone to bed. Suddenly, I was frantic to do a breast self-examination. I was forty-eight years old and had never had such urgent feelings before. From where had this thought come? How many other women were doing self-exams on New Year's Eve? Were you? There it was, a hard lump in my right breast. I could palpate it between two fingers. I knew that most lumps were benign, but a very close friend had passed away from breast cancer eight years earlier. She told me she had turned over in bed and felt the lump and knew immediately that it was cancer. Did I somehow know the same thing? No, I could not discern any such message.

Early on January 2, I made an appointment to see my gynecologist, who ascertained that there was indeed a lump. He asked me if it hurt, and I told him there was no pain at all; he appeared to be concerned with my answer. He made an appointment for me to see a general surgeon, and, within a few minutes, I was sitting in the surgeon's waiting room. Thoughts were racing through my head. I knew that the majority of breast cancers did not hurt and that the majority of benign lumps were tender, but there are always exceptions to every rule. I was trying to remain calm. My last mammogram had been the previous May, and it had been negative.

I had a needle aspiration of what turned out to be a cyst filled with liquid and blood. My breast then felt normal. There was no sign of the cyst. It had disappeared as if by magic. This was on Friday; by Sunday night, the lump had returned. Because of the speedy return and the blood in the cyst, the doctor recommended a biopsy.

I was due to return to my surgeon for the results the following Friday, but his office called to say he had to go out of town—could I come in on Tuesday? I smiled into the telephone and said yes and thought, what a flimsy excuse. Why didn't the secretary just ask me to change my appointment if someone else needed that time? The real reason I was asked to come in early never crossed my mind.

"The test results show a malignancy in the wall of the cyst."

There it was. I had cancer. *Cancer,* the word my father could never say out loud, as if it tempted Providence to voice the name. Don't panic. Pay attention to what your surgeon is saying. DON'T PANIC. Breathe slowly, try to concentrate. He said I had a choice of a lumpectomy or mastectomy; both, in his opinion, were equally effective. Because of my friend, I knew if I ever had breast cancer and had a choice, I would choose a lumpectomy.

"Now that I have said all this, I know you haven't taken it all in. Why don't you go home and call for another appointment? Discuss this with your husband; take the time to come to a decision you are happy with. If you like, we can schedule the operation for this Thursday."

This Thursday! Surely people do not make such hasty decisions. But some do. I had heard of people opting for immediate surgery; they cannot wait to get rid of the offending body part. Because I had read various articles over the years, I knew that I had time to make an informed decision. I wanted the very best for myself.

The nurse gave me a nice hug and told me that she knew I'd be okay. Hugs are absolutely wonderful when they are genuine. I felt the tenseness and stress flowing away and was left with a feeling of calm, the strength gathering again. The nurse's father had died of breast cancer in 1978, so this was a disease she was very aware of. Approximately 1,400 men are diagnosed and 260 die each year of breast cancer.

I fled the doctor's office and drove home, my thoughts in a frenzy. Finally, I turned into my driveway. Oh, to be in one's own home, one's own sanctuary, a buffer against the outside world. I called Ray, my husband. Please, please, let him be at his desk. "Ray Duda," he answered. The relief flowed through my body.

"Ray, it's Loraine."

"Hel-lo," he said in that special way of his.

"I have just come from the doctor's office, and it isn't good news. I have breast cancer."

There was a brief silence and then he said he would like to go with me to talk to my doctor and see what my options were. A plan of action! Something to arrange! Thank goodness! It seemed as if my brain was working in slow motion.

My body and me—we had shared so much and done so much and come through so much together. Now we had to face breast cancer together. Would it be insurmountable? I didn't think so—tough maybe, but not impossible. Nothing is impossible. I was a four-pound premature baby born in wartime England, which in itself is an accomplishment. I was born fighting.

I went to see an oncologist and another surgeon for a second opinion. Each time a friend went with me—a very good idea, because even though I had my list of questions, I seemed to miss some points in my anxiety. I remember the surgeon swinging back on the little hard chair in the examining room, templing his fingers, and saying if it were his wife he would recommend a mastectomy. Thank goodness I was not his wife! In all fairness, he did tell me that in my case either mastectomy or lumpectomy would be a good choice, and, in fact, people who had lumpectomies had a slight edge over those who had mastectomies.

I talked with several people who had breast cancer, although it was difficult to find someone who had chosen lumpectomy. I became a frequent visitor to the library, and I usually left with an armful of books.

A friend told me that a friend of hers had had a mastectomy with immediate reconstruction and thought this the only way to go; she had been delighted with the outcome. For a while, I toyed with this option before I remembered that my decision was firmly lumpectomy—I was so stressed out I almost changed my mind!

What really added to my stress was the medical insurance company. My husband had started a new job just the month before I was diagnosed. Every bill, every request was returned with the response, "You have a preexisting condition." It took many, many telephone calls and hours that turned into months to get all the bills resolved. My surgeon explained to the company that since I had not had the disease before, it could not be a preexisting condition, and he wrote a couple of letters to them on my behalf.

I made the decision to have a lumpectomy followed by six weeks of radiation. A date was set for surgery, and I started the usual battery of tests.

Now that my decision had been made, there was one more very important thing to do—tell that wonderful, unselfish, loving being, my mother. My mother lives in Perth, in Western Australia, the other side of the world. I am an only child and very close to my mother. She is now alone, my father and her brother having passed away. I wanted to make everything as easy for her as possible. I telephoned a friend of hers, and she agreed to be at my mother's house when I called. I also made the airline reservation for her; her flight was scheduled to arrive the day after my surgery.

S-day arrived, and Ray drove me down to the hospital, armed with a stack of magazines to read. Ray is uneasy in hospitals. When he took me in for the biopsy, he was so agitated he could not wait in the private room with me but moved to the main waiting room. One assumes that it is harder for the patient than for the family members waiting outside, but this is not always so.

The surgery went well, and my dear husband was waiting for me in my room. For my hospital stay, I had bought some satin pajamas, and what a blessing they were. One can slide and glide over the sheets when turning over with ease and minimal discomfort, nothing has to be pulled over one's head, and the small drain can be easily pinned to the waistband of the pants. The drain is a small tube coming out of the armpit with a small, soft bulb on the end that has to be emptied a couple of times a day. This is painless and easier to handle than it sounds. I went home with mine, and the doctor removed it in his office a few days later.

The morning after my surgery, I noticed that when I lifted my right arm, there were two strings that popped up along my forearm. They were not painful, but I could not imagine what they were. It was not until I started an exercise class that I found out that they were nerves. With exercise, they did disappear. This was the day I met my oncologist for the first time. He discussed my radiation treatments and told me that after that there was no need to see him again unless I felt the need to or had any questions. I felt really good about that; obviously, he was not concerned, so why should I be?

Home! Home! Home! How good it felt to be back. Ray dropped me off and then had to go to the airport to meet my mother. What her thoughts had been on those long flights I could only imagine. I ran down to the garage to greet her, and she was so surprised to see me home and dressed.

My mother went with me to the hospital for my radiation orientation. I was mapped with a marker pen, asked not to wash it off the first night, and then had my tattoos, which are tiny dots. With my freckled skin, they are not noticeable.

Someone had told me that they had been in a very small room for their radiation treatments. As I am a little claustrophobic, I was apprehensive, but the room turned out to be large and airy, with bright, colorful prints on the walls. What a relief! The hardest thing to do was to try to get my right arm above my head. Although I was still doing my exercises, that problem persisted; I did not have full range of motion.

I underwent five weeks of radiation, followed by one week of booster. I scheduled my appointments for lunchtime and worked just half a day because I wanted to see my mother and I wanted my body to be as rested as possible. It seemed as if I was always leaving work late, driving to the hospital in a rush, and then hurrying to the radiation unit. In hindsight I would schedule more time for this so as to arrive in a calmer state of mind.

The radiation went well until the fifth week, when, after my treatment, I was walking to the elevator and felt as if a huge weight was pressing down on me. This must be how a deep-sea diver in a suit feels on dry land. The pressure felt so unbearable, I was afraid my high heels would snap! After this, I stopped wearing high-heeled shoes and started wearing flats. The pressure started to dissipate with the end of the treatments, but it is only now, after nearly five years, that I am thinking of buying some shoes with heels again!

I had never sunbathed in the nude or used a tanning booth, so the skin on my breast was very white and unblemished. I did get a sunburn and a few extra freckles from the radiation. Fortunately, before I started to blister or peel, the treatments were over. The sunburn and freckles have long since disappeared. The red area was larger than the area mapped by the tattoos, especially over the top of the breastbone near the neck.

I have always had what I thought of as immature breasts—very soft, with no firm shape. My radiated breast was now very firm. After approximately two years, my radiated breast became soft again, and I now have a matching pair, except for the nipples—the radiated one is lighter in color.

The back of my arm is still numb, and I need to shave only half of my underarm. At first I had to be careful about digging in the garden, as my thumb and first finger would throb and then start to swell. This was mild lymphe-dema. I found if I sat with my elbow resting on the back of the sofa and my hand resting on the wall behind, the swelling would dissipate. Sometimes, if I raised my arm straight in the air, fingers pointed, Ray would clasp my fingers with both hands and, grasping tightly, draw his hands down my arm to my shoulder. This was great; it really helped reduce the swelling and took away the bloated feeling. I still do not hike or walk with my hands hanging down; I usually put my hands in my pockets.

In one of my support groups, I met a woman who also had a lumpec-tomy followed by radiation. After about three years, she noticed a pimple-type lesion on her shoulder. This turned out to be angiosarcoma, a rare cancer of small blood vessels and soft tissue. She had surgery, followed by several courses of very intensive chemotherapy through an IV at home. Angiosarcoma is a radiation-induced cancer. Neither she nor I were advised of this possible outcome from radiation. When she complained to her doctor, she was told it did not usually show up for about ten years. Be forewarned!

While undergoing my radiation therapy, I found an announcement for an exercise class at a local hospital, specifically for women who had breast cancer. I immediately started going to the evening sessions. It was a fabulous class. It did not matter how you looked or how well you could do the stretches. Everyone there had been through what you had been through and was very understanding and encouraging. It was great to be able to discuss problems and fears and swap helpful information. We did special stretches that helped get the full range of motion back in the afflicted arm. One exercise was espe-cially helpful:

Lie flat on your back, hands by your side, holding a yardstick. Lift the yardstick upwards, in an arc toward your head, as far as possible. At first you may have to stop when your arms are straight up in the air, but as you push a little, gravity will take over, and your knuckles will eventually touch the floor. You will feel a z-i-i-i-p as though a zipper has opened; I thought I had either hurt my arm or ripped my shirt. But in less than a week, I had full range of motion back.

The exercise class stopped, due to lack of funding. To continue our exercise program one of the women and I started to walk every Wednesday evening. We walked in rain, snow, or sunshine. Because we could not take estrogen, we started to get worried about osteoporosis, so, after two years of walking, we started working out with weights at a body-sculpting class for women.

After about a year, I noticed a minor discomfort in my left hip, which became more pronounced over the months. Three miles into a hike, this pain would kick in; every time I got into bed, I would feel a twinge; the first few steps I took after sitting for a while, I limped. Of course this worried me; the fear of metastasis is always present. I had various tests and X-rays and a bone-density test, which showed I was losing some bone mass in my left hip. One of the doctors mentioned that I could try physical therapy, since this might be bursitis. I jumped at this and went for six sessions over a period of two weeks. They heated me up, showed me stretching exercises, and iced me down. I followed these exercises for two months and am happy to report I am now pain free. I also started taking the new drug Fosamax to build up my bone mass. I find it hard to believe that even though I work out with weights twice a week and hike two to four times a week or snowshoe once or twice a week, my bone density is below average. I will take the Fosamax for a year and then decide what to do.

One of the side effects of not taking estrogen is hot flashes. I have had them for three years. So far, I have not found anything to relieve them. I am lucky to live in a dry climate because the perspiration evaporates in a few minutes; when on vacation in a humid zone, there is no such relief. On the plus side it is wonderful to feel great every day and not just one to two weeks a month—no PMS anymore!

In the fall of 1993, I went to Washington, D.C., to participate in a march to the White House, organized by the National Breast Cancer Coalition. This was one of the most wonderful, inspiring days of my life. People were cheering us on and waving, traffic stopped, taxi drivers were smiling and honking to give us encouragement. President Clinton promised us $400 million. What a high I was on! I became close friends with the local women I traveled with. How wonderful to have friends with whom you can discuss your innermost fears, the newest information on breast-cancer research, treatments, and many other related subjects. One's other friends can be very sympathetic and caring, but unless they have gone through a life-threatening experience, it is not the same thing. I still see friends from one of my original support groups, too.

A couple of months later I was in Las Vegas looking at the newly opened Luxor Hotel. Remember the $400 million we were promised in Washington and that we had worked so hard to achieve? Well, I read that this new hotel, a place for frivolous entertainment, had cost $400 million to build. What I had considered a large amount of money was just enough to build this hotel! I looked at the building and saw a stylized breast growing in the desert, instead of an Egyptian pyramid. There was an intense beam of light thrusting upwards from the nipple into the starry heavens and beyond. Is this our beacon of strength and hope for the future to those who will follow?

Where does breast cancer come from? This is a question we ask ourselves over and over. No one knows, and every year there seems to be a new thought on this issue. I cannot help feeling that pollution and the chemicals with which we surround ourselves and smother our food have some bearing on cancer. I am also a strong believer that we have not heard the last of the secondhand-smoke issue. Do our lifestyles and environments contribute to breast cancer or is it something we are born with that just waits for the right circumstances to start to develop? There is some wonderful work being done with the breast-cancer gene, and this is marvelous for the few who have breast cancer in their family. The treatment for everyone is still barbaric.

What about my own environment? For the first five years of my life, I lived just outside London; back then there were days in the winter when we did indeed have pea-soup smogs. Then my family had a sheep farm in Western Australia for a few years. There was no pollution in those wide-open spaces; we were about two hundred and fifty miles from the city of Perth. After that, we moved to Jersey, in the Channel Islands, between England and France. Yes, this is where the Jersey cows come from, and the milk always had a good three inches of rich cream on the top. There is no industry in the islands and, therefore, not much pollution. I do not remember the farmers using chemicals on their handkerchief-sized fields; in fact, many of them still fertilized with seaweed. I moved to London to become a flight attendant. I often wonder if I was exposed to harmful rays while flying, but I have not heard that flight attendants have a higher incidence of breast cancer. Lastly, I moved to the United States in 1971, living first in the south, then in the west in an exceptionally clean city.

In 1982, I started taking aerobic classes and was influenced by the writings of Covert Bailey and other writers on health issues. Even though I was not eating a high-fat diet, I eliminated some more of the fat from my meals. As a child, I was used to eating one or two very thin slices of meat and two or three vegetables for my main meal. I ate very few fried foods, an occasional fish and chips being the exception.

I have always felt that diet is a very important ingredient for a healthy life. What we put into our bodies must surely make a difference to the outcome. I now feel that with the population explosion of this planet, it is impossible to raise enough food without artificial means, and good nutrition has fallen by the wayside. So much of our meat and poultry appear to be saturated with antibiotics and hormones to try to fatten the animals for market. Daily, I take vitamins C and E, selenium, beta-carotene, and calcium.

When friends at my supper club asked what they could do, I requested that they make me a dish with beta-carotene and bring the recipe with it. That way, we all gained something; it was a learning experience for us all!

There has been some controversy about wine being one of the causes of breast cancer. The French and Italians drink a lot of wine, yet I have not heard of a higher incidence of breast cancer in either France or Italy. I feel, therefore, that a moderate amount of wine is not the culprit. Jersey is only fourteen miles from the French coast, and most of us grew up drinking French wine.

Has breast cancer made a difference to my life? Yes!

I am nearly five years out, I feel great, and my energy level is high. Having breast cancer is not something I would have chosen, but it is another facet of life I have experienced and has molded me into the person I am today. I definitely feel stronger through having had this experience. At first I could not think of the future beyond the immediate day or two; to think of retirement or some trip six months off would send shivers down my spine. I did not dare to plan so far ahead. Finally, I feel comfortable enough to make plans for the future. I want to pack as much as I can into each day and do all the things I want to do. Ray tells me I cannot have and do it all, but I disagree; I am going to try. I have a new motto: Today is the day and the time is now.

I would like to leave you with two thoughts:

1. You are very special.
2. Life! Be in it! (an Australian expression)

Facing Metastasized Breast Cancer

We all know it can happen. We wake up in the night knowing that a few cells could have escaped our efforts, could be out there doing their damage. This chapter tells how those women to whom it did happen faced, and are facing, the reality of metastasized breast cancer.

The first part of "A Raft in the Ocean" was written before the metastasized cancer was discovered; the author chose to add to her essay rather than revise it when she found the cancer had spread. The author died before publication of this book. Her story details the importance of support groups, especially for patients with metastasis. It also expresses her rage at the lack of sufficient research and the uncertainty about the best ways to treat the disease.

Like the first story, "These Are my Bonus Days" was also written in two stages. In this case, the second stage describes the author's bone marrow transplant, which has given her new hope for a longer, pain-free life.

The final story details a couple's fight with their insurance company to provide the wife the treatment she needed to stay alive—a fight that may have cost her her life.

A Raft in the Ocean

Beverley Seale

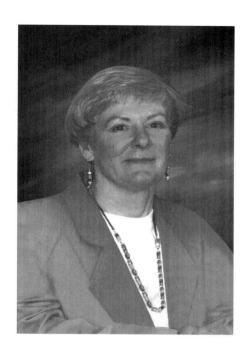

Beverley was born in Montreal, Canada, the eldest of four children. She moved to the United States in 1966. She was the mother of three boys and grandmother to four grandchildren. Until her disability retirement in 1991, Beverley worked as an assistant in obstetrics/gynecology and dental and oral surgery. She particularly enjoyed traveling; participated in skiing, swimming, aerobics, and reading; and loved being with family and friends.

Medical Bio

In May 1988 Beverley had her annual physical examination and was advised to have a mammogram. At this time, a nurse discovered a lump; the subsequent mammogram showed a suspicious density in the central portion of her left breast. That same afternoon, her surgeon confirmed the presence of a 2-centimeter firm, mobile mass, which was also associated with slight retraction of the skin. A fine needle aspiration cytology confirmed the physical examination and mammographic suspicions that Beverley had a breast cancer. Because of the proximity of the mass to the nipple, and the associated skin retraction, the decision was made to treat her with mastectomy rather than breast conservation. A subsequent left modified radical mastectomy with immediate subpectoral prosthetic reconstruction was accomplished. Eight of the twenty axillary lymph nodes showed evidence of metastatic breast cancer. After her surgery, Beverley underwent radiation therapy, and, because her tumor was estrogen-receptor positive, she was started on Tamoxifen. Following the completion of her radiation therapy, she experienced some contracture around her breast prosthesis and underwent a revision of her reconstruction surgery.

Beverley remained well until the fall of 1991, when she began experiencing pain in the left hip. An evaluation by her oncologist revealed the presence of metastatic breast cancer in the left hip bone. She underwent radiation to the area of cancer recurrence with an excellent clinical response.

When Beverley's mammogram revealed the presence of the suspicious lump, her previous mammograms were reviewed; this retrospective review revealed that her breast cancer was visible on a mammogram taken a year before the malignancy was discovered.

I can remember someone asking what it was like to be told that one has cancer and to go through the experience. For me, it was the most lonely time in my life. I felt that due to circumstances beyond my control, I had been placed in a rubber raft without oars or a rudder, to be tossed on the waves in the middle of the Pacific Ocean, with the instruction that I was to get to shore—a rather awesome task at the beginning. The human spirit is not frail, and hindsight tells me that I came through that journey without too much difficulty. I have landed in a new world, one that is full of excitement for me, and I am viewing it with rested eyes. I truly have been given a second chance, and the second part of my life is of better quality.

. . . .
What a difference a day makes

On the Friday morning before the Memorial Day weekend in 1988, I went to have my annual mammogram. There was no reason for me to be apprehensive about this examination. After all, it was only nine months since my last one, and I had had an exam two years before that. They were both clean and clear, and there was nothing in my genetic background to concern me. Breast cancer was unknown to all the females on both sides of my family, back to my grandmothers. Well, my education on breast cancer was about to begin.

During the physical part of the examination, the nurse very quietly and discreetly brought to my attention an indentation in my left breast. After the examination and X-ray, I stayed until the technician was happy that good X-ray results had been obtained. I was told to get in touch with my doctor later that afternoon because the radiologist would probably be calling with information. I was surprised rather than frightened, still not thinking that this could be a malignancy.

When I called my doctor, she asked me what had taken place that morning. I told her, and she replied that she would contact me again within thirty minutes. Ten minutes later, she called to say that she had made arrangements with a surgeon to see me in less than one hour. Was I able to go?

The surgeon was concerned with the indentation of the left breast, and we agreed that he would do a needle aspiration with results available later the same day. He was able to obtain some fluid. He then told me that the indentation was a definite sign that it was probably breast cancer and that the fluid he was able to aspirate would either confirm or deny suspicions. He gave me a rather quick lesson in the biology of breast cancer, and we decided to make some decisions based on the assumption that this would be a positive result. I remember telling him that whatever he recommended, I would be very happy to do. He said he didn't work that way, that it was my breast and I had options as to how I wanted this handled. He would be glad to do whatever I chose.

I very quickly made the decision to have a modified radical mastectomy. There was never any hesitation. The fact that I could have a cancer in my body frightened me terribly, and I wanted it removed, along with as much tissue as possible around the tumor. I didn't want to take any chances. I also decided to proceed with an implant at the time of the surgery. I was not depressed leaving his office. I really felt good about the decision I had made, and I was happy with my surgeon. So I returned to work.

Later that afternoon, he called to say that the laboratory had confirmed his suspicion; what were my wishes? We arranged for me to go in on Wednesday for surgery that afternoon.

By the time I returned home from work that Friday, I was emotionally exhausted. After supper, I called my three sons to let them know what was taking place. I had held together exceptionally well since early that morning, but after calling the children and reassuring them that everything was going to be fine, it was time for Mother to fall apart.

Cancer is a very frightening word. We seem to hear it connected most often with the dead rather than with the survivors, but I found it very hard to see how this could possibly be a death sentence for me. I tried to figure out how I could have gotten myself into this predicament. I had kept my weight under control, eaten three good meals a day, gotten anywhere from six to eight hours of sleep, made sure I always stayed physically active, and enjoyed all kinds of sports. (On the other hand, I had been a smoker for thirty-eight years. I quit immediately.) Other than a broken leg from skiing, a tonsillectomy at age thirty-four, and occasional bouts with flu, chest cold, or head cold, I had always considered myself in excellent health. How could somebody possibly have a cancer growing in her body when she felt as well as I did? It was then I realized I was not in control of my life. Here I was, fifty-six years old, living alone, supporting myself (a new experience of a year and a half), my children living out of the state, my immediate family—mother, sister, and brothers—all living in Canada. Somehow I was going to have to get myself through this.

I telephoned my three closest friends and shared this news with them. They were concerned, sympathetic, and supportive. We all knew how serious this disease can be. A year earlier we had buried a very close friend who was only thirty-two years old.

That Memorial Day weekend was not a fun time. I spent most of it walking. I am sure I walked thirty miles in those three days, and I cried buckets of tears trying to grasp the situation in which I found myself. Life couldn't possibly be ending for me at such an early age. After all, Mother was eighty, still going off to Europe every year for an extended vacation. There was no reason for me to believe that I would not follow in her footsteps. The possibility of dying before the age of eighty-five was something I had never considered. Well, one is never too old to learn something new.

After three days of wallowing in self-pity, I decided how I was going to handle this. I was going to be tough, I was going to be self-reliant, I was going to fight my way through it. After all, it was my life, and I wanted every day coming to me. That was my approach, and I am still working on it.

I took a couple of hours off work on Tuesday to have a bone scan done. The doctor was very pleased with the results, and my attitude was a little more upbeat.

On Wednesday I checked into the hospital shortly after noon and was very relaxed going into the surgery later that day. Once in the operating room, I felt that the operating team were friends who would take care of me. I went to sleep very easily and woke up the same way. My hospital stay was short and pleasant, with slight discomfort, but nothing I would call pain. When my family picked me up the day I was released, we went to the park for lunch. It felt so good to be out in the fresh air and have the grandchildren running around.

I did not go to work the following week. The next Wednesday, I called my department head to let her know that I was getting along well and looking forward to coming back to work the following Monday. I mentioned that I was not sure the doctor was going to let me return to a forty-hour week during the first week, and I was shocked when she said that I had been hired with the understanding that the job required forty hours a week and that was what she was expecting. I was very upset by the remark. I wondered how anyone could be so insensitive, but the message came through loud and clear about what I was going to need to do to keep my job.

A day or two later, I went to the doctor's office to have them check the dressing and to get the pathology reports. I was unprepared to have his assistant tell me that the tumor was an infiltrating ductal carcinoma, approximately 2 centimeters in size, and that eight of twenty nodes were found to be positive. I remember feeling that I was passing on a horrible thing to my children and grandchildren, and that upset me greatly. Now I knew that I was in for some follow-up treatment, probably chemotherapy, and with all of the horror stories I had heard, I wondered how I was going to be able to get through that.

This latest news was more than I could handle. I felt like I was going to go crazy if I didn't discuss my feelings with someone who could understand what I was going through. At that time, I knew only one woman who had had this disease, and she had not lived two years with it. I called the American Cancer Society to see if they would put me in touch with someone with whom I could discuss my fears. They found a woman in my neighborhood, and I was invited to her home. She was very kind and took the time to sit down with me. However, I felt she had little understanding of my situation; she was a woman in her early eighties who had gone through breast cancer twenty-five years earlier and had had no node involvement. I felt somewhat better after leaving her house, but I was really unable to communicate with her or even make her understand why I was so upset. Somehow, the end of that day came, and I got through it. It was a very lonely weekend for me, and I was delighted to return to work on Monday.

. . . .
Who's in charge here?

That week when I saw the doctor, we discussed what my follow-up treatment would be. He had presented my case to the tumor board, and they had recommended that I be a candidate for chemotherapy, so he was sending me on to an oncologist. By the time I had the appointment with the oncologist a week later, I had accepted the fact that I would be on chemotherapy, that it would be unpleasant, but that I would get through it. Losing my hair was not something I was concerned about; being physically ill did concern me. My job was my livelihood, and I wondered how I was going to do both the job and chemotherapy.

The oncologist asked me if I knew why I was there; I said that I had been told I was a candidate for chemotherapy as my follow-up treatment.

He asked where I had gotten that idea, and I told him that my surgeon had presented my case to the tumor board, and that was their recommendation. He said he did not agree with what the tumor board had decided and that he must not have been in attendance when my case was presented. Therefore, he was taking it back to the tumor board, as he felt radiation was going to be better for me than chemotherapy. So everything was put on hold again for a few more days.

The oncologist eventually called to say that he had presented the case and the tumor board had agreed that radiation was the treatment of choice. That made me wonder if any of them knew what they were doing. Could the tumor board change their minds in less than two weeks? How were these cases decided, how were they presented, who presented them, and were the patient's best interests being looked after? Who was looking after my best interests?

I fought the radiation all the way through. It was a very unpleasant experience. Because of the fairness of my complexion, I figured that radiation was going to burn and perhaps even blister me. But I knew it had to be done, so I presented myself for tattooing on a Monday, with treatment the following day.

When I saw the thickness of the lead shield that had been made for me, I realized what a dangerous procedure this was. I found it to be very scary but painless. After the second treatment, the radiologist told me he was unhappy with the results they were getting; he was sorry, but they would have to re-tattoo me the following day. I was extremely upset. These people were experts—why weren't they doing it right the first time? Why were decisions being changed from chemotherapy to radiation? This was my life that they were changing their minds about. I was really wondering who was in charge here and if anybody really understood anything. That is when I decided that I needed more information

I went to the library and checked out books on breast cancer. My reading has never been more intense than it was in those days. The more I read, the more I felt that nobody really had a solid answer for breast cancer. I also realized that I was going to need some help to get through this whole experience. The doctor's assistant suggested that I get in touch with the YWCA, which had a program called Encore. All of the patients in the group were breast-cancer patients. Meetings were held once a week at the YWCA, and I found that meeting with these women and listening to their stories advanced my education greatly.

Besides the group conversation, the program included simple floor exercises and pool aquacise. Three weeks postsurgery, I was given permission to start both. I could see weekly improvement in arm motion, and it was very relaxing for me. I looked forward to our weekly meetings.

I went for my second tattooing and continued with the radiation. I changed the treatment times to 7 A.M. so that I could be at work by 8 A.M. without anyone knowing that I was into secondary treatment. I was able to get through the five weeks of radiation. I felt very strongly about this because I did not want to have people going out of their way to treat me differently. The only change I had to make at work was to sleep on my lunch hour; otherwise, I would not have been able to put in my forty hours. Because I was so tired after work, I ate most of my evening meals in the cafeteria at the hospital, came home, opened the mail, and went to bed. I was exhausted and slept almost ten hours nightly.

During radiation treatment, I again felt like I was totally out of control and was going to end up in a mental hospital if I didn't get a better handle on what was happening. I told the doctor's assistant I needed help, and she wondered if I would see a psychiatrist. I didn't hesitate. For approximately six weeks, I went to see a wonderful woman who helped me get back on track.

By the time I reached the last week of treatment, my skin was quite badly burned; it was exceptionally dry, had cracked in a few places, and bled. It also became difficult for me to swallow, and I was given a liquid to drink thirty minutes before meals so that my throat would be numb and I could swallow without pain. That worked very well, but all of my meals tasted like peppermint.

On the day of my last treatment, I was told that the doctor was very happy with the results he had achieved with the radiation and that it would indeed be my final treatment. That was by far the best news I had received in the last two months. I remember leaving the hospital with tears in my eyes. I had made it through my most difficult period of breast cancer. During the next few weeks, I continued to treat the burns I had received, and each week I felt a little better, a little stronger. My spirits started to rise. I had had to give up the Encore group when the radiation burns became uncomfortable; now I returned to the group and participated in the discussion and the floor exercises.

Once I had finished peeling, front and back, it was time to do something good for myself. I started swimming three times a week, rather timidly at first because I was hindered by range of motion. But that soon returned, and within a very short time I was lap swimming. That was one of the best things I did for myself. Now that I was feeling better physically and emotionally, and enjoying my swimming activities, my mental attitude was on the upswing.

With my radiation treatments complete, I once again presented myself to the oncologist. Because my tumor had been an estrogen-positive receptor, my follow-up treatment at this time was hormonal therapy. I am taking Tamoxifen daily and doing fine.

. . . .

Coming to shore

My recovery started the day I was diagnosed because the surgeon was forthright, giving me the negative and the positive sides of the disease and asking me how important my life was to me and how hard I would fight for it. He made me realize that this was not going to be minor surgery and that my life would never be the same. The quality of my recovery would be up to me. He told me that I could get through this alone, and I believed him. But I was not alone. I had the doctor and his assistant to keep my spirits up. I had three wonderful friends who listened to my fears and anxieties. The support group at the YWCA played a big part in my recovery.

I have learned that I am only partially in control of my life. I no longer take for granted that I will live another thirty years, but I've made some changes to make that goal more likely. I stopped smoking. I continue to eat three meals a day, with little or no junk food, but each meal is nutritionally balanced. Vitamins are an important part of my daily routine. I am much more aware of stress, and I do my darnedest to control it. I am convinced that stress plays a big part in breast cancer, so I do not put myself at risk.

I'm also more attentive to my body and the implications of seemingly unimportant things. For example, two or three years before the diagnosis, I had periodic itching in my left armpit—not a surface itch but something deeper. I now know that this is a possible signal of trouble. But it would never have occurred to me to mention this annoyance to a doctor.

The very worst part of breast cancer is the psychological impact that you must deal with on a daily basis. There are daily reminders of what has happened to you—in the shower, when you are getting dressed, when you reach for something on a high shelf in the cupboard. This constant reminder makes me very aware that I must get the most I can out of every day, and many times that entails just looking at the flowers, watching the leaves blow in the wind, seeing the sunrise or sunset, tasting good food, and really being aware of my senses and surroundings.

I still consider myself in the recovery process and hope to stay there the rest of my life. Each day gets better and I now have an inner peace that I never had before. I walked into the surgeon's office that Friday morning as one person, and by the time I left that office I was a totally different person. Something very special happens to some people who have this disease; there is an electricity in these women that I have found nowhere else. They are upbeat, positive, and in charge. I believe that, like myself, they are living each day as if it were the last.

Recurrence is a possibility for me, but it is not something I dwell on. Should it happen, I will deal with it, and until it happens, this is the best time of my life.

I have one strong desire that is yet to be fulfilled; however, I am working on it. I feel a commitment to all women to educate them in the prevention of breast cancer and the management of their treatment if they do develop it. I also want to offer all the support I can to the new groups of women who are experiencing this. I believe that support groups, properly run, are the best way for women to face the reality of breast cancer and come through it in a healthy manner.

I now know that medicine is practiced by human beings, not miracle workers, and they are not infallible. They do the very best they can with their present knowledge. I feel I am in very caring hands with all of my doctors. However, from my contact with the women in my support group, I know that many medical professionals treat their breast-cancer patients in a very condescending manner. Women need to be given information and have some say in their treatment. They have a right to honesty, a right to an answer to a question, a right not to be told, "Leave that to me; I will worry about it." Women are losing part of their sexuality with this disease, and too many doctors are saying, "There, we have taken care of that, go home and get on with your life." If only it were that simple. We need to educate women to take the initiative, to ask hard questions, to get answers, to be responsible for themselves.

We also need to vastly increase the research on the causes and treatment of breast cancer. AIDS is getting most of the media attention and research money right now, even though about one-tenth as many people die of AIDS as die of breast cancer. However, we know how to prevent AIDS from spreading and how to avoid contracting it ourselves. No one has yet told me what I did, or did not do, to contract breast cancer. Research needs to be done to give us some answers. If the men in this country were losing a testicle to cancer at the rate that women are losing a breast, I think we would have an answer by now.

. . . .
A second voyage

Sometime in March 1991, I was seated on a chair at work. As I stood up and took the first step, my left leg gave out, and I thought I was going to fall. I said, "You silly girl, you are far too old to be working on your feet full-time, and your leg is letting you know that it is tired." I regained my balance and went on with my day.

In April, the same thing happened. I went to take a step and felt as if my left leg was going to give out. I had an oncology appointment in May, and when I saw the doctor, I told him about it. He did a lot of thumping and banging and twisting of the left leg. This caused no pain, so he felt that it was probably an arthritic condition. I was happy to accept his word.

I immediately made plans to return home to eastern Canada during the first two weeks of July. I had not visited my family for fourteen years and felt that it would do me a lot of good. In the meantime, I had my annual visit with the surgeon, who found no problems at all.

However, sometime after the fifteenth of June, I did notice that this condition was getting to be a nuisance. My leg was continually giving out, and I was never too sure when it would happen. I realized then that I had a problem that needed to be attended to, and I was concerned that I had metastatic disease. But I also realized that if this *was* metastatic disease, I could not go home with this weighing so heavily on me. I would not want to share the information with my family. I went and had an absolutely marvelous visit—it did me a world of good.

While on vacation, I noticed that I had difficulty getting out of a car. I needed to hang onto the door to lift myself up. It seemed to be getting from a sitting to a standing position that was my problem, rather than walking.

When I returned home, I went to my internist. An X-ray of the hip and pelvic area came back and the diagnosis was that I had degenerative arthritis, indicating that at one time I must have had a severe blow to the hip area. I didn't remember this ever happening, so I found it hard to accept. But I thought, "Okay, it sounds logical that a sixty-year-old woman could be starting to have arthritic conditions." When ten days of antiinflammatory drugs produced no results, I was given a different drug, again for ten days, and again with no change.

At this point, I went back to my oncologist and asked for a bone scan. It showed a "hot spot" on the left femur. Again, it was possibly an arthritic condition, but the oncologist recommended an MRI, so I had one immediately. Yes, there was a 2-centimeter tumor on the bone. I immediately started two weeks of radiation.

I stayed at work but had a lot of pain. Partway through the radiation, I realized I was not going to pull this off without people at work knowing what was going on; already people were suspicious. I was told by my personnel department that breast-cancer metastatic disease was definitely a cause for disability retirement. I also applied for Social Security disability. Both of the disabilities were very quickly approved; thirty minutes after I handed letters from my doctors to my employer, the federal government, I was dismissed. I was sent home and told not to come back. I was absolutely overwhelmed at the speed with which things *can* work in government!

Due to insurance problems, I had to change oncologists. I found this very unnerving, as I had been with my oncologist for over three years, and we had a good rapport. Fortunately, I found a new one, and I am absolutely delighted with him. He has a much more liberal approach to the disease and does not make me feel that I need to come in every two or three months to be checked. He feels that I am intelligent enough to contact him if I have a problem.

I had no problems from the radiation, except for extreme pain for four to six weeks, which was very debilitating. However, the radiation oncologist assured me that the pain would leave eventually, and it did. My bone has healed beautifully, and it's solid. If I care to go skiing now, I can.

One Sunday in December, I started to turn over in bed and found I could not do it. I had extreme pain in my chest. I had no idea what was going on and was very frightened because I live alone. It took me about ten minutes to roll out of my bed, as the pain was so excruciating. Not thinking too clearly, I decided to wait until morning before I did anything. When I did call my doctor, he said, "Quickly call 911 and get yourself to the hospital. We'll be waiting for you." The paramedics arrived less than three minutes from when I called. They did an EKG in the house, connected me to an IV, and put me on oxygen immediately. In the meantime, a friend passing by on her way to work came in and took over for me. I felt she was a guardian angel in my time of need. She stayed at the hospital all day.

After numerous tests, they diagnosed a pulmonary embolism. I still had some residue in my leg, and the blood clot was in the left lung, which is why the pain was so excruciating. I sat in the hospital for a week. I requested no visitors and no telephone calls. I did not feel like talking to anyone. I felt that my first job was to get well, and I didn't need to play hostess and entertain people. This annoyed some of my family and friends, but they have to understand that I know what is best for me. Finally, I am learning to take care of myself.

I was sent home, and I have not had any serious problems as a result of this incident. The doctors feel the problem is not cancer related; I have a family history of phlebitis, so this is probably a hereditary condition.

Now, at the end of January 1992, my life is clicking along very nicely. I am enjoying every day. I plan to do some traveling, probably monthly, anywhere from California to who knows where in the world. I attend a support group for metastatic breast cancer patients on a weekly basis. It is called The SOUP Group—Supportive Outreach with Understanding People. This is the one place we can talk about our treatment, our innermost feelings, and our innermost fears with a group of people who totally understand. Healthy people do not understand, nor do they want to hear anyone talk about dying, and each one of us knows we are dying. It will be in different stages and in different ways, but certainly our days are numbered. Since the time I joined, we have lost two members—this is a very unforgiving disease.

In 1991, I requested copies of all my mammograms from the radiology department. I looked at them myself, and even without a medical background, I felt that I could see a very distinct "something" on the 1987 mammogram that turned out to be a more defined circle in 1988. I consulted a lawyer; he felt that an error had been made in 1987 and that I should have been brought back for a second mammogram and perhaps even a biopsy. I feel that the mass *was* visible in 1987, and I have requested that a malpractice suit go forward. I will not settle out of court. I want this to go to a jury trial.

I pray that I will live long enough to see this come to a conclusion. It will not change my life at this point. The die is cast for me. But perhaps it will change a procedure. Perhaps there is not enough time taken in reading mammograms; perhaps they are read at a time of day when the radiologist is tired. We are told to have a mammogram, but we need to be able to rely on the person who reads the mammogram. If an error was made, and if, as a result of this malpractice suit, procedures are changed so this doesn't happen to anyone else, then I will feel the contribution of my life to cancer will have been to a good purpose. I will not have died *only another* victim of cancer.

. . . .

A third voyage

In August 1993, I looked at my someday-I-would-like-to-do list and decided to become a certified scuba diver at age sixty-one. The sport has brought me a new circle of friends, travels to exotic places, and a view of another dimension of God's planet, possibly the most silent and colorful.

By March 1994, I was in pain and suspicious of more disease to the bone. A bone scan was done, and I again underwent two weeks of radiation to the left side of the pelvic bone—after two tattoo sessions. Then I developed pain that caused me to limp on my right side. Another bone scan was done in August that revealed five hot spots, three on my ribs and two on the right side of the pelvis. This was puzzling and was presented to the tumor board. The consensus was to maintain the status quo to give the new medications a chance to lay down new bone. The limping and pain continued for a few months, then disappeared.

I developed blood clots again in the leg. I am on blood thinner and probably will be for the rest of my life. Today, in mid-1995, I am detecting bone pain in new places. I have requested tests be done, and perhaps there is another voyage ahead of me.

Life is uncharted territory. It reveals its story one moment at a time.

[Beverley died on October 12, 1995. In a deposition taken as part of her malpractice suit, her radiologist admitted he was negligent in missing the mass on her 1987 mammogram. A subsequent ruling by the supreme court in Beverley's state will serve to extend the statute of limitations for seeking legal recourse in cases involving a negligent delay of diagnosis.]

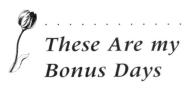

These Are my Bonus Days

Doreen Weyland

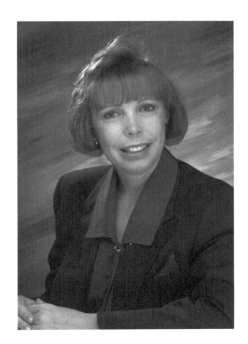

Doreen has received her paralegal certificate and POST-certificate for category II police officer training. She currently works for an international law firm while attending night school to obtain her bachelor's degree.

Doreen's life has greatly improved since her bone marrow transplant. She now concentrates her efforts on reducing stress and enjoying life (especially with her nieces and nephews).

Medical Bio

In January 1988 Doreen discovered a lump in her left breast. Her gynecologist subsequently confirmed the presence of the 1-inch lump, and a mammogram was obtained. The X-rays showed findings suspicious for breast cancer, and her bone scan showed a small focus of potential metastatic breast cancer in her fifth thoracic vertebral body. Doreen elected to proceed with breast-conservation therapy. During her surgery, the lumpectomy portion of the operation demonstrated multiple areas of invasive breast cancer within the specimen, indicating that breast conservation did not offer the best option for control of her breast cancer, and, intraoperatively, the decision was made to proceed with a left modified radical mastectomy with immediate reconstruction. She made an uneventful recovery from surgery, but subsequent pathologic evaluation of her lymph glands revealed that three of the sixteen nodes removed contained metastatic breast cancer. By the fall of 1988, the area of question that had been discovered on her initial bone scan did prove to be metastatic disease to her bone. She has gone through courses of chemotherapy and radiation therapy, as well as the surgical removal of her ovaries.

Because her metastatic breast cancer continued to progress and because she was having constant pain from the involvement of her bone, Doreen elected to undergo autologous stem cell harvest and high-dose chemotherapy. This new treatment appears to have resulted in a dramatic suppression of her metastatic breast cancer, and, at this time, Doreen shows no evidence of residual breast cancer. She is looking forward to the completion of her breast reconstruction.

When I was growing up, I believed that doctors knew everything. Throughout the last four years, I have been rudely awakened to the fact that this is not true.

In January 1988 I was busy sewing a wedding dress, veil, and line dresses for my brother's fiancee and her attendants. I had also begun to sew the spaghetti-strap dress that I would be wearing to the wedding. As I was trying on my dress to mark the placement of the straps, there it was. I remember thinking that this was not a lump, but in the back of my mind and in the pit of my stomach, I knew this must be what a lump would feel like. I had no idea what was in store for me.

After panic and hysteria set in, I telephoned a good friend of mine who was just finishing her residency in obstetrics and gynecology. Instead of the calm, sensible person I pride myself on being in a crisis, I became a stupid, frightened, and numb person. I later realized that in the next year and a half I chose to remain numb.

On the advice of my friend, I called my gynecologist the following Monday morning. I was quite surprised that they were able to get me in that morning. After an examination, I had a mammogram. Looking back with 20/20 hindsight, I remembered that in October 1987 I had commented to my gynecologist that the color of my left nipple had changed and did not match the color of my right nipple. I had also stopped perspiring under my left arm. He said he did not notice any color change and that people sometimes stop perspiring anyway. I truly believe that these were my first warning signs.

At 3:30 P.M. that same day, my gynecologist called me at my office to tell me I had an appointment with a surgeon at 4:00 P.M. I wanted to yell at him that he had said this was probably nothing. The impact of what was going on slowly began to hit me.

. . . .

I never dreamed it would be cancer

After the examination, the surgeon asked that I get dressed and come to his office to talk. It is not every day that you suddenly find yourself face to face with a doctor you did not choose who is about to change your life.

My surgeon explained that after looking at my mammogram and performing the examination, he was 99.9 percent sure that I had breast cancer. I don't know what I was thinking up to that point, but I never dreamed that it would be cancer. He explained to me that he wanted me back in his office Monday morning to discuss the various options. I was so anxious that I wanted to discuss it right then, but as he correctly surmised, I was in shock and would not have remembered very much of what he said.

My surgeon arranged a meeting the following day with two of his patients who had gone through a mastectomy and a lumpectomy respectively. You don't know how much it helped to have someone (still alive) tell me about her experience with cancer. They even offered to show me their scars. This was very funny to me, and I thought, "Is nothing sacred?" Later I would be offering to do the very same thing for a newfound friend going in for her mastectomy.

I decided on a lumpectomy and six weeks of radiation treatments. Within two weeks of that fateful Saturday night, I was to be operated on. Before the operation, I had a bone scan to see if there was any metastasis of cancer. Unfortunately, my scan reveled two "hot spots" (possible cancer areas), one on the fifth thoracic vertebra (T5) and one on my right kidney. I had to go back to the hospital the day before my surgery for more X-rays. They flushed my kidney and did another X-ray, and then it no longer appeared as a hot spot. The radiologist said he would not try to biopsy T5; the only way to safely biopsy T5 without the risk of hitting the spinal cord was to open the chest, move the heart and lungs, and go in from the front. This was not an option! They would only have done that in a life-and-death situation. His final diagnosis was that I had a fifty-fifty chance that the hot spot was a bone island rather than a cancer spot. My doctors kept telling me that when breast cancer metastasizes, it rarely goes to only one spot, so my chances were good that T5 was only a bone island.

Friday was the operation. My surgeon told me that it should only take a few hours. The only thing I was concerned with when I woke up in the recovery room was what time it was. I had gone in at noon and my doctor told me it was now 8:00 P.M. I knew something had gone wrong—and then he told me he had had to do a mastectomy. I found out later that there were two additional tumors under the one they knew about, which is why they performed a mastectomy. My surgeon chose to begin reconstruction at the time of the operation, so I had an implant when I awoke.

....

The chemotherapy machine

When I first heard of chemotherapy, I really had no idea what it was. I envisioned a huge machine, much like a CT Scan, in which you would lie. It would inject this chemotherapy. It was a big relief to find out that it would consist of injections in the doctor's office. *Chemotherapy* is only chemical therapy.

Based on my receptor test, my oncologist recommended a combination of drugs consisting of Cytoxan three times a day; prednisone three times a day (to be reduced at the end of the six-week period); an injection of fluorouracil; and an injection of methotrexate. Treatment began in March 1988. Every Friday I would stop at the hospital on my way to work and have my blood drawn. I had decided to schedule my appointments for my injections at noon on Friday; that way, if I were to get really tired and sick, I would be able to go home and rest for the weekend. By Friday night, it was all I could do to drive home and get to bed.

I was pleasantly surprised the first few weeks on chemotherapy that I was not throwing up continuously. I was, however, nauseated for six months. I remember wondering if I would ever feel good again. At the beginning, knowing I would do this for one year, I thought I would never make it. Having my face double in size due to the prednisone and watching my weight increase daily didn't help. Still, I knew I had to eat well; I believe that I would not be alive today if I had not eaten as well as I did. In my mind I envisioned bad cancer cells eating away at me. As long as I kept creating healthy cells, then the bad cells would not have a chance to overtake the good cells.

Living on my own, I was able to rest often without having to worry about any commitments. Most of my friends knew that I was unavailable from Friday to about Tuesday of the following week. Once we had an idea of how the drugs were affecting me, my oncologist suggested that I take my treatments in the middle of the week so that I could enjoy the weekend. That turned out to be a great suggestion. I could feel lousy at work and be on the upswing by the weekend. It turned out that it did not matter when I had my injections because the prednisone turned me into an insomniac. I was wired and strung out, and I was existing on two or three hours of sleep. And, of course, for the twenty or so hours I was awake I was eating my little heart out. My surgeon made me feel a little better by telling me he had never seen a fat terminally ill patient. That was great—permission to continue to eat.

While coming off the prednisone, life was horrible. I remember crying every time I had to look at my face in the mirror. My eyes were just slits in my head, and everything was so swollen. I had to hold up my eyebrow to put on eye shadow. The thing that hurt the most was that everybody would tell me I did not look any different. I guess people don't realize that you can see what they can. I was very fortunate in that I did not lose all of my hair. My hair thinned about 30–40 percent, but I never had to use the wig I purchased the week I started my chemotherapy.

Well, as it turned out, I only had to endure the chemotherapy for six months. I was scheduled to leave on a vacation to South Carolina when I started having chest pains. My oncologist, the hospital radiologist, and my surgeon diagnosed me as having an enlarged heart. However, the heart specialist said that I had a minor problem with one of my valves. He felt that that was not the cause of the chest pains. My oncologist stopped all of my chemotherapy. I found out later from another doctor that I probably had a toxic reaction to the amounts of Cytoxan I was taking.

It was time to repeat the bone scan to see if there were any changes. On the way to my oncologist's office after the scan, I told myself that the spot on my back was not cancer, and, if it was, I would just go on to the next step. I was very composed while I waited for the doctor. He started by telling me that the scan indicated the spot on T5 was larger and that the conclusion was that it had, in fact, been cancer. Then he told me that my right pelvis showed some tumor activity. He kept on talking to me, and I kept on asking questions. I was okay until he said, "Do you understand what I am telling you?" Of course I did. It was the opposite of what I kept praying would happen. I would die from this disease. The scan also told us that the chemotherapy was not working. Damn! Can you believe that I was nauseated for six months and it did not even help contain the cancer?

. . . .
The radiation machine

About a month later, I began to have a lot of pain in the area of T5. The pain was a burning, aching pain, and I could not sleep. The decision was made to begin a series of radiation treatments on the T5 area. I would have to go to a different hospital, and I had to try two radiologists before I felt good about one. If you learn anything from my story I hope it is this: if you are not comfortable with your doctor, then CHANGE. When it comes to cancer therapy, I must trust my doctor.

Toward the end of my radiation treatments, I began to experience a pain in my throat. There were times during the night when I would wake up and not be able to breathe. The pain seemed to increase over the weekend, and I was not able to swallow or eat. When I spoke to my radiologist, he indicated that because they were radiating over my esophagus, the lining would be irritated. He gave me some medicine that numbed the throat so I could eat. Well, the medicine worked—not only did it numb my throat, it numbed my tongue, lips, and taste buds. Once I finished my treatments, my throat improved, but I still have a problem when I try to clear my throat. Obviously, this was caused by the radiation. When I suggest this to my doctor, he looks at me like I am crazy. I think we patients know more about our bodies than our doctors do.

....
Change of life at thirty-two

Next I started hormone therapy. I began with a drug called Tamoxifen. Everything seemed to be in check until mid-November, when I began to feel extremely tired and just not right. I talked with my oncologist about my symptoms, and he felt that the hormone treatment might not be shutting down the ovaries. The ovaries are the largest producer of estrogen in a woman's body; estrogen feeds breast cancer, which is why they try to stop its production. I decided to have my ovaries removed (oophorectomy). The Monday before Thanksgiving, I was in the hospital for my surgery. After I recovered, I felt great. It seems that the ovaries had been functioning all along, so I felt that having the surgery was the right decision.

I had decided only a year before this dreadful disease that I really wanted to have a baby. But having my ovaries removed and not being able to bear children became secondary to staying alive.

But I was not prepared for hot flashes! Going through the change of life at thirty-two was not my idea of fun. Looking back, I should have consulted a female gynecologist because I think women are more sensitive to the whole issue of hormones.

In March 1989, I continued to have pain in my back, and the decision was made to radiate T7 and T10, where the bone scan indicated I had two new tumors. This sent me back for another round of fifteen radiation treatments. By now I was a pro going back to finish a familiar battle.

Near the end of these radiation treatments, I began to experience more nausea and some really bad headaches. I told my radiologist about this; he said he was leaving town for a few days, but to let the resident know if my symptoms got any worse. When I spoke to the resident, saying the symptoms were about the same, she revealed that they thought I had a brain tumor. She told me I needed to have a brain scan done that day. I was really afraid that I was dying. After I had the brain scan, I waited anxiously for my oncologist to call me with the results. When he called and said that everything was fine and that the scan showed no sign of brain metastasis, I cried with relief!

When my radiologist returned, I told him what had transpired and that if he was ever suspicious of something as serious as a brain metastasis, then he had better discuss it with me. He said his resident was a little overzealous. However, the price of agony, dollars, and time spent worrying was not worth one overzealous resident.

Because I had needed more radiation, my oncologist felt that the Tamoxifen was not helping control the cancer. The next treatment to try was a hormone called Megace. I began taking these pills in July 1989, and after about six months, I knew something had to give. This hormone made me a totally unreasonable person. After a continuous, month-long headache and ongoing depression, I went to see a neurologist, who prescribed some anti-depressants for me. They seemed to help.

. . . .
How much pain does it take?

The Megace helped me through the next year. However, I was begin-ning to have increased pain again and consulted my oncologist about my options. I was under the impression that there were many more hormones to try. But I found out that I had only two left. This news hit me smack in the face. I asked my doctor why he had never explained that there were only a few hormone options. He became quite angry and started to lecture me about not abandoning a treatment unless it was truly necessary. I asked *him* to explain to me how much pain was sufficient to warrant a new hormone; he continually berated me because I could not explain to his satisfaction the extent of my pain.

The next hormone I tried was amenoglutethimide. This hormone basi-cally shuts down your adrenal glands (situated on top of both kidneys), which produce some estrogen. I had to supplement this hormone with a low dose of prednisone. Even with the low dose, I still put on some weight, which depressed me. But my feeling now is that if something is keeping me alive, I need to quit complaining about it. Sometimes that is easier to say than to live!

This hormone treatment's success makes me very mellow—something new for me! I am enjoying life more than I ever have. I have learned to appre-ciate true friendships and discard the superficial ones. I find joy in spending time with my two-year-old nephew. He has sweet, unconditional love for me. I try to keep a simplified mind-set. I believe that anxiety and stress played a large role in my developing cancer in the first place.

I have spent the last year and a half with a support group for women with metastatic breast cancer. Studies have shown that women who are involved with support groups live an average of eighteen months longer than women who are not. I am counting on this! I have received more information on breast cancer and cancer treatments from the women in this group than from any of my doctors. I am finding out that not all doctors believe in treating breast cancer the same way. There are some doctors who will not stray from conventional textbook treatments; they ignore the research being done in universities around the country. I found out that my oncologist was one of these. Needless to say, he is now my ex-oncologist.

I consulted with my current oncologist regarding his feelings about using experimental treatments, and he agreed to help me with whatever treatments were reasonable. We obtained information from other doctors regarding new advances with Autologous Bone Marrow Transplants. I decided to try whatever was available to keep me alive.

. . . .
The bone marrow transplant

In October 1991 a very dear friend began a bone marrow transplant for a sarcoma in her leg. I met her doctor, and, over the next few months, I spoke to him about the possibility of undergoing a peripheral blood stem cell transplant, an autologous transplant (one for which you are your own donor). After an examination and several hours of being educated about this procedure, I gave the consent for the initial submission to my insurance company.

To my surprise, within three weeks my insurance company authorized this procedure. Most insurance companies decline to do transplants for breast cancer because they claim that the procedure is experimental and investigative. Yet the courts have determined this procedure to be a proven treatment. The sad thing is, most people do not know they have recourse when their insurance companies decline. There is now a national network of attorneys who offer free legal services to people who have been turned down by their insurance companies for transplants for breast cancer.

We decided that I would begin the process of harvesting bone marrow on March 9, 1992. There are two harvesting methods. The first is the traditional method in which you are given a general anesthesia and approximately five one-inch incisions are made across your hips. They insert an instrument through the incisions that attaches to the hip bone and allows a needle inserted through this instrument to extract marrow. About two hundred extractions of marrow are made, which are then processed and frozen.

Because of my marrow involvement, I was only a candidate for the second method of harvest, called pherising. This method involves a very different procedure. I would begin with a short hospital stay to have a central line

(Hickman) put in my chest and receive a high dose of chemo. Tubes would extend from my right shoulder and chest area. The Hickman is very important because it allows the doctors to administer all of the chemo agents and drugs necessary during the transplant.

I was admitted to the hospital on Monday morning to have a Hickman put in. After the surgery, I was taken to my room, where they started a very large dose of Cytoxan. It only took about three hours for the Cytoxan to enter my system, but I was to remain in the hospital until Wednesday morning to be monitored and to keep the fluids going through my system. The chemo drugs are very hard on your organs, and they must keep fluid pumping through you so the drugs do not have a chance to destroy any vital organs.

As I was talking with the doctor who would be conducting my pherising, I started to get extremely sick, and, before I knew it, I had passed out. I was only out for about thirty seconds, but because of this episode I had to undergo a night of CT scans to confirm that this was not a seizure and there was no cancer in my brain.

After receiving instructions on how to care for my central line, I was released to go home. The one shot of chemo I was given would get my counts down close to zero, and then I would be given a growth factor (GM-CSF) to raise my white counts rapidly. After my counts were up, they would begin the process of pherising.

The process involved returning to the hospital every day for five to ten days to be hooked up to a machine that extracts your stem cells out of the blood. The machine takes the blood from your system through one of the tubes on the central line, spins off the stem cells, and returns the rest of your blood to you through the second line. It took about four to five hours a day. There is virtually no pain involved; I would just lie in bed and watch television or read a book. The end product of this five-hour session is very small but very valuable.

The theory behind pherising is that when they drop your counts to zero and then administer the growth factor to get your counts up rapidly, the new, immature stem cells that begin to grow are believed to be cancer-free. These cells are extracted before they have a chance to be attacked by the cancer so that when they are transplanted back into your body, they are cancer-free. Because they are your own cells, your body will not reject them. Amazing!

The period during which the chemo knocks your count down is a dangerous one because your body is so susceptible to infection. By getting your white counts back up, the growth-factor drug helps to shorten that period of susceptibility. I felt fortunate to have completed the pherising in five days.

I then had to wait for a bed in the transplant unit to become available. They have rooms with special air-flow systems designated for bone marrow transplants. You are not allowed to leave the room once you begin your transplant and cannot receive any flowers or anything that would contain bacteria. You are advised not to have many visitors and those who do come must wash their hands and put on gloves. No one is allowed skin-to-skin contact with you. You take every precaution conceivable to avoid an infection.

I believed that I would have to wait three weeks for a room, but it turned out that I waited only three days. Once there, I began with four days of continuous chemo. During this time, they are also pumping a lot of fluids through you to protect your organs, so, naturally, you have a catheter. With the catheter at one end, my central line (both tubes) connected to chemo, and two IVs in my hand (because the surgeon inserted the wrong type of central line), I was a human pin cushion (and I use the term *human* loosely)!

I slept a lot during this time; it was not until after the chemo was finished that I became terribly sick. It took over a week and a half to come up with the right combination of drugs to ease my nausea. This was a difficult time, because it is hard to concentrate on getting well when you are nauseated and vomiting.

One of the side effects from the chemo is mucousitis. This is very annoying! The lining of your gastrointestinal system is irritated, you develop sores in your mouth, throat, and nose, and you cannot eat. I was pretty fortunate in that I only suffered with this for about a week.

After the four days of chemo, they give you a day to rest! The actual transplant is on the sixth day, when you receive your marrow/stem cells back through the central line. They had ten bags of cells to give back to me. The procedure required about ten to twelve doctors, techs, and nurses and took about twenty minutes—most of the time was spent going through the precautionary checklist to make sure the stem cells were mine, not someone else's.

Now the waiting game, the counting of days until you graft. You are grafting when your counts start to come back, and I was told that it would take up to three weeks. I told them that I would graft in three days, and they did not believe it. But I knew when I was grafting one night because I had a great amount of pain in my tumor areas. When the doctors made their rounds that night I told them I was grafting, and they kind of smirked at me. Well, the next morning they were not smirking, they were smiling—I had grafted in six-and-a-half days!

Now that my counts were coming back, I began to get restless. Finally, twenty-one days after entering the hospital and fourteen days posttransplant, I was discharged. When I returned home, I just sat outside on the back porch.

It was so nice just to get some fresh air again after being in the same room for so long. It is amazing how much you take your freedom for granted until it is taken away.

I had to follow up at the clinic three times a week after I left the hospital. Whenever I was out and around people, they requested that I wear a mask. I also had to stay away from small children because they are walking cultures and always have a sniffle or cold. At home, I had the walls cleaned and the house dusted, and I found a special antibacterial soap to wash the vegetables in before cooking them. They told me to defrost meat in the refrigerator and not on the counter; make sure everything is cooked well-done; avoid having flowers or plants in the house because of the bacteria in the dirt; and stay away from pets, public restrooms, and public telephones. I became afraid to even touch my face without first washing my hands with antibacterial soap.

After I was one hundred days posttransplant, the restrictions were relaxed. Actually, I followed most of the restrictions only for about three weeks. When my counts stayed up, I figured my immune system was starting to work again. And I stayed on prophylactic antibiotics.

I am now back at work full-time and just happy to be alive. When my co-workers said it was good to see me, I responded with, "It is good to be seen!" I have such a better outlook on life now. For four-and-a-half years I did not make any long-term goals or plans because I knew that I did not have long to live. Now I sometimes get overwhelmed with the knowledge that I can think about a future and make plans. I am very excited that I will be here to watch my nephews grow up. It's satisfying to know that I do not have to work in any position that does not benefit me and utilize my skills.

I do not take this Pollyanna attitude to the extreme. I know that there is a chance that I can have a recurrence. But at least I get to spend this time pain-free and daring to dream. People always tell me that they could never have done this, but I tell them they would be surprised at what they can do. Until you are tested, you do not know what your limits are. I wanted to live; I did not like the alternative to not fighting for what I wanted. For once, my aggressiveness paid off in a big way.

. . . .

On staying alive

When you have cancer, having an oncologist that you trust is crucial. I called several friends in the medical field and inquired as to the best oncologist in my city. I have found a team of two doctors that best fits my needs. I know that they will be by my side fighting with me, and, if I lose, they will be by my side holding my hand. You cannot ask for more and you cannot accept less.

The most important message to all women is that early detection can save your life. I was too young to be considered for a mammogram; I found the lump myself. If I had not taken action as soon as I found the lump, I would be dead today. I used to feel that they should lower the recommended age for the first mammogram. However, after attending a seminar on breast cancer, I learned that the density of breast tissue makes it almost impossible to detect most tumors any earlier.

Breast cancer is not just a woman's disease. It affects everyone. Most people do not know that one in two hundred men also get breast cancer every year (compared to one in nine women*). I know that new breakthroughs being discovered will help all cancers. We need to get involved in our treatments and demand to know what they are doing to our bodies. The archaic treatments we are receiving are almost as deadly as the cancer itself. I know that if the cancer does not kill me, the effects from the treatments will shorten my life through heart disease, lung disease, or radiation-induced cancer.

Today we have some new drugs to help with nausea and to help build your white blood count; we have new painkillers and we have bone marrow transplants. However, we still do not have any idea what causes breast cancer. We need to find the cause and the cure. I am participating with my community to increase the awareness of breast cancer. I will march and protest if I have to. I do not want to be one of the 44,500 women who die every year from breast cancer.

If we do not demand the money for research from those in Congress who control the purse strings, then we might as well just put our heads in the sand and die. That would make it very easy for the men on the hill, but this is one time that I will not take the easy way out. I demand my rights as a human being. I cannot sit by quietly and watch as thousands of women die each year. I will work for our welfare as long as I can breathe. I only wish women ten years ago had taken a stand; maybe the cause and cure would have been found by now. Maybe it will take electing more women to Congress to ensure our interests are represented.

My oncologist has always told me that "the only predictable thing about breast cancer is that each case is so unpredictable." I know now that I can handle anything. What is bigger in life than being terminally ill? I am now five years LUCKY in life. These are my bonus days.

----

*The current (1996) statistic is that one in eight women will have breast cancer.

The Cindy Friend Story

Randall R. Friend

Cindy was a beautiful young wife and mother with hopes and dreams much like ours: graduations, weddings, grandbabies, and growing old with her husband, Randy. Because of a strong family history of breast cancer, her surgeon performed a random biopsy and found cancer. What followed was a bilateral mastectomy, six months of chemotherapy, and a belief that she would never have to worry again.

But within two years the cancer had spread to her lungs. Her passion for life was so great that she chose to have a bone marrow transplant.

It was a miracle—she seemed cured! But just before her six-month checkup, a nagging cough started. The transplant had failed. Though Cindy never gave up hope, she died eight months later.

Cindy started to write a chapter for this book but was unable to complete it. The following are the thoughts and ideas that she intended to share:

"Every day, in every way, I am getting better and better."

These are the words I live by. They mean everything to me as I live my life ten minutes at a time. No one knows what tomorrow will bring. I feel that I've been to hell and I'm back to tell about it. I have been to the edge, faced the fear head-on, and am stronger because of it.

On a warm Wednesday in June 1990, my world fell apart. I thought I had pneumonia and found out it was tumors on my lungs. My physician asked me to go to my oncologist and have him look at my X-rays. Fear sets in, and you want to believe he is just being overly cautious. But no, he's telling you in the most delicate way that there's something wrong, seriously wrong. I thought I had won the battle with breast cancer after I had had both breasts removed and six months of chemotherapy. It had been an accident, after all, that my doctor even found the lump, and, because of a family history of breast cancer, recommended that I go through the chemo. I thought my life was on the uphill climb and had been for one-and-a-half years.

My oncologist informed me that the breast cancer was back and in both lungs. I was devastated. I felt the need to scream, to be angry, to run. I felt that I needed to go back to bed and get up again, that this wasn't really happening. But it was. He informed me that with a little luck, I had a year, maybe a little more—a very bleak outlook. I left his office in complete numbness.

I drove as far as my old place of work, where my good friend was working, and asked her if she had a minute to talk. I totally fell apart. I'm not sure why I stopped to tell her, but I guess I felt a need to tell someone. She drove me home, and we went to my husband's place of work to tell him. This is probably one of the hardest things I've ever done, with the exception of telling my children that I had been told I was not going to live. I called my sister Linda to tell her and to ask her to tell my other brothers and sisters. Emotionally, I had had it.

Linda has also had both breasts removed because of cancer, as had our mother, who died at the age of forty-nine in 1973. Linda called back to say that her doctor had encouraged her to tell me about a new procedure called bone marrow transplant. They have been doing it for only five years but have seen some remarkable results. Oh, the hope this gave me.

Cynthia Jo Friend
March 20, 1953–July 8, 1991

. . . .
The story begins

Cindy loved wild purple flowers, autumn days, summer nights, Harley Davidsons, and, for reasons I never fully understood, she had an unconditional and uncomplicated love for me. No matter what stupid or crazy scheme or plan I came up with, Cindy supported me all the way. She was a doer, a friend; she was my wife. She never disappointed, never broke another's trust; you could count on her. She could make a truck driver blush and inspire an angel to sing. You always knew exactly where you stood with her; she simply wouldn't tolerate any bullshit. Her priest called her "wonderfully irreverent." She was the only true constant in the universe.

With the national divorce rate exceeding the 50 percent mark, our marriage was the stuff poets write about. All she wanted from life was to be with me. And all I needed was to be with her. She was my bride, my lover, my best friend. She possessed uncommon charm and grace and an indestructible spirit. She could laugh—and did laugh—when there was nothing left to laugh about. She had a contagious love of life. Neither one of us was completely whole without the other. The times we were together were the best times. I never realized how much she meant to me until I was losing her. There is no way anyone reading these words can appreciate what I'm trying to say unless they've had the distinct pleasure and honor of knowing her.

Cindy was a victim—a victim of a disease that stalked her relentlessly and eventually consumed her; and a victim of a system that places corporate profits ahead of human life, a system dedicated to pricing the human soul.

Her story—our story—begins only a few years ago. Due to a strong family history of cancer, the specter of this enigmatic illness loomed over her head day and night. Her mother had died in her forties from breast cancer, and her older sister had already weathered one attack of the disease. Familial cancer can progress in several directions: it can jump a generation, genetically fade itself out, or be persistent and tough. No one can ever predict its course. Though she never faltered, never showed fear, Cindy carried this worry with her much of the time. We would talk, of course, about the chances of her getting cancer, but our twenty years together had been so full, and we had already survived jobless times, a near-fatal illness of my own, raising two wonderful children, Matthew and Melinda, and so much more. It did not seem possible that we would be forced to face cancer.

Faith and hope are blind, and they blind those who believe in them. Still, something inside Cindy, an instinct perhaps, knew. And when her sister had a second occurrence of breast cancer, Cindy knew something might be wrong with her too.

Cindy knew a dynamic doctor, a friend, who had been doing research in precancer diagnoses. He thought that there might be a way to spot cells changing before they become cancerous. Although he felt that Cindy was in no immediate danger, at her request he agreed to do a biopsy and see if there was a change in her cell structure. Cindy was afraid, but she had to take control of the situation, and she felt that this was the right direction to take to save her life. On the day of surgery, he selected a random spot to biopsy.

The procedure was simple and uncomplicated, but this was one of the worst days of our lives. In a matter of minutes, the doctor met with me in the waiting room and informed me that he had chanced upon a pea-sized tumor. My world was twisted out of shape; reality was unacceptable. A person's mind tends to go numb rather than face what it is unable to deal with at the moment. The doctor stayed only a minute, and I was forced to face the evil truth alone and unarmed. I remember little except that I paced back and forth over and over again. I refused to believe what I had been told.

Cindy accepted the news like a general reading a battle report. If she was afraid, she did not show it. We knew that no matter what the bad news was, statistically early detection is a good thing in treating cancer; that was the lifeboat of hope to which we clung. Though we had not gotten the news we had wanted, we had firm ground on which to fight the enemy. The doctor, Cindy, and I later discussed what the best course of action might be and decided that a bilateral modified mastectomy was the only safe thing to do under the circumstances. Again, it was not what we wanted, but it was the best action to take. Cindy was scheduled for surgery as soon as possible. We decided that reconstructive surgery with breast implants would be done as well.

The time between diagnosis and surgery was short but hard on our emotions. Her surgery this time was much longer. The hours passed slowly in the waiting room. The doctor believed in doing all he could now rather than scheduling follow-up surgery later. So he did the reconstruction at the same time he removed Cindy's breasts. Over seven hours of worry later, his nurse came out to tell us that Cindy's surgery had gone well and she was doing fine. I was even able to see her for a moment or so. I felt good and desperately believed that everything would be all right now.

After a short stay in recovery, my Cindy was able to come home. She was strong and very positive about what had happened and about the future. Her lymph nodes had been cancer-negative, which was very good news indeed. Her recovery was rapid, and marked the beginning of the very best time in our marriage. She was advised to go through six months of chemotherapy just to be sure, and again we decided it would be worth it.

Chemotherapy is nearly as bad as the disease. It is a form of treatment that nibbles away at a person's dignity. But Cindy was strong and suffered through sickness and hair loss with a joke and a smile. She never submitted to either the cancer or the cancer treatment. Six months went slowly for her, for us, but it, too, came to an end, and the future looked bright once again.

We entered a period in our lives when we had so much to be happy and thankful for. In celebration, we decided to build our dream house, the one we had been working towards for more than sixteen years. We visited model homes, pored over house plans, and even toyed with house designs of our own. We selected a building lot and a builder, and we were on our way. This was going to be Cindy's house in every way.

Cindy worked out, went running, and grew stronger and stronger right before my eyes. She thrived on watching her home grow. Every night after work, we walked from the house we were renting to the new house to see the progress and plan a future that was going to be sublime.

Our new home was nearly, if not completely, perfect. During the next year, we grew even closer together and more in love. We seemed to be in a pattern of happiness now, and nothing dared go wrong.

Then Cindy developed a persistent cough. There was a particularly bad bug going around at the time, and we thought she had caught it. Still, the cough hung on and on. I was at work when Cindy went to see our family doctor. He thought at first that it might be pneumonia, but he was not sure, so he asked her to seek another opinion from her oncologist. The news plunged us back into the nightmare. Cindy was told that her condition was not pneumonia. It was breast cancer that had metastasized to her lungs.

This time it was even harder to accept than before. Our life together was working happily—it just was not fair!

Cindy's oncologist told her that she had a year to live, maybe two. I don't know of anything harder to accept. The kids and I were consumed by fear and anger; we shouted, we cursed, we cried, we wanted to attack a faceless enemy. Again, Cindy was strong and more concerned about those she loved than about herself.

. . . .

The insurance nightmare

Cindy's sister told her of a remarkable procedure called Autologous Bone Marrow Transplant, ABMT for short. The idea was that although chemotherapy was an effective treatment for cancer, the chemo was nearly as hard on the patient as it was on the cancer cells. In particular, the patient's bone marrow dies quickly during chemotherapy treatments. This prevents the ideal amount of chemo from being administered.

With ABMT, some of the patient's bone marrow is removed, harvested, and frozen in liquid nitrogen. Then the patient receives as much high-dose, potent chemotherapy as he or she can take, in the hope that all of the cancer cells will be destroyed in the process. Such a high dosage would normally cause death, but then, at the end of treatment, the patient's healthy bone marrow is reintroduced into the system, allowing the system to recover. Many other forms of cancer, such as leukemia, have been successfully treated in this manner. Preliminary results from this treatment had been impressive; patients given a year to live were surviving for three or more years without a recurrence. Only time would call it a cure, but for us it was such a delicious hope. Even failures in the program were given another two or three years to live.

It did not take much discussion to decide that we were going to see if this could be done for Cindy. She talked to the head of the ABMT on the phone at length, and we flew to Iowa as soon as it was possible.

During the examination and review of Cindy's records, it was clear that she was an ideal candidate for ABMT. One big problem raised its ugly head, however—money! An ABMT is very expensive—one hundred to one hundred and fifty thousand dollars. And the hospital made it very clear that it expected the money up front. When I asked about the Hippocratic oath concerning the ethics of turning away a person in need of medical treatment because of a lack of funds, I was told without emotion or apology, "We aren't turning patients away; we're just taking those with money first." This was to be the first bitter lesson in modern medical and insurance ethics (using that word loosely).

At the time, we were not concerned. Cindy and I had always provided for ourselves, never needing nor asking for help. We worked for what we wanted and needed, and we had the very best medical insurance you could get, or so we thought.

Because payment had to be guaranteed before admittance, Cindy and I had to return home to arrange the finances. We believed at the time that there was not much required in the way of preparation. Our insurance company, part of a national insurance giant, required that we call and get preauthorization, but that was expected to be routine. Unfortunately, when we called them, they were vague and indecisive about giving us a preauthorization. At the time, I felt that it was inconceivable that anyone could, with a clear conscience, turn someone down for critically needed medical treatment.

After a lot of calls, they did give us an answer: they said no because they felt that ABMT was experimental and exempt from payment in accordance with the benefit plan. At first we were numb with shock. We were insured—how could they turn us down? Then there was a lot of anger and fear. That weekend was emotional agony, but on Monday, they called back and said that they were going to reconsider. Hope restored, we were deceived into believing that we would get the medical treatment Cindy needed to live.

The next Friday, they told us once again that they would not pay for ABMT treatment. Another bad weekend. The very next Monday, they called back to say they were going to reconsider. This pattern went on for more than two months. We pleaded with them to at least make up their minds. People and organizations had come forward offering to start a fund-raiser but could not do so until the insurance issue was settled. At one point, a representative called us and, in confidence, advised us to get an attorney.

Cindy and I were both guilty of being too trusting and perhaps a bit naive about the ways of the world when it came to money. It never occurred to either of us that the insurance company would really deny authorization for medical treatment, committing the moral equivalent of premeditated murder. Still, slowly a veil was lifted, and we saw the ugly, lethal side of for-profit-only, corporate America. I got busy and wrote to my congressional representatives. I called anyone who might be able to help, including the governor.

In the meantime, we hired Cindy's family attorney to look into the matter. He compiled an inch-thick package of information proving that ABMT was a legitimate treatment for breast cancer and that the company was obligated to pay for the treatment. The attorney was able, after much coaxing, to get the company to put their denial into writing. When the written refusal came, he countered with the evidence package.

Under the federal insurance system, if there is a difference of opinion on a problem such as ours, the Office of Personnel Management (OPM) is supposed to arbitrate each case and settle the issue. Our attorney contacted OPM and sent them the document package. (It was also sent to our congressional representatives.) Our attorney was confident that the insurance company would agree to pay for Cindy's treatment. He gave them time to look over the package and tried to call them. They refused to talk to him or to us. Our attorney advised us to seek local legal counsel and file suit against the company.

In the meantime, more than three months had passed, and we were running out of time. For someone given only a year to live, those months spent fighting an insurance company were a criminal waste of time. Cindy was on conventional chemotherapy, but she could not stay on it forever. If the cancer spread to her bone marrow, the ABMT could not be done. Meanwhile, a fund-raiser had been started in case we could not get the company to reverse their decision.

We talked to a local attorney; he carefully looked over our documents and, after unsuccessfully trying to reach the insurance company himself, decided to file suit. After five months of delay, a lawsuit was filed, giving the company three days in which to make a decision.

The fund-raiser had collected enough money to pay for the bone marrow harvest, so Cindy and I decided that it would be best if she went back to Iowa City to have that done before it was too late. I had to stay home to work and care for the children.

While this was going on, the press got wind of our story and did several articles on our plight. Many of the local television stations also ran stories on us. Even some Iowa City newspapers and television gave us coverage. This generated substantial support for us. Of all the government officials contacted for help, only one senator responded to our request. The OPM ignored us and our attorneys. Months later, the OPM supported the insurance company's position, citing the National Cancer Institute (NCI) and the American Society of Clinical Oncology (ASCO) as organizations calling ABMT experimental. When I contacted NCI and ASCO, they denied ever taking a position of any kind on ABMT with the OPM. For whatever reasons, the OPM fabricated information sources at a terrible cost to Cindy and me.

. . . .
The ABMT treatment

Because of the lawsuit, the insurance company gave in at the last possible moment and agreed to cover the ABMT. Cindy was in Iowa and I was at home, but our joy and relief carried over the miles. Our lawyers told us that we had to drop the suit and pay our own attorney fees. We agreed, of course.

One down side was that the attorneys' fees had consumed nearly all of the money donated up to that time. It bothered me, and still does, that money given towards medical treatment had to be used to pay attorneys to get what we were legally and morally entitled to. However, the situation had snowballed to such a point that we had little control anymore. And the money did get us medical treatment, albeit indirectly.

I was able to travel to Iowa just before Cindy was to go in for the ABMT treatment. It was not easy to face what was ahead, but it was clearly our last and best hope. Already, nearly five months had been wasted, time that should have been spent in ABMT treatment. The doctor was still positive, and, though he would have preferred to have started earlier, he felt that the treatment still had a chance to be effective.

We spent the day before her admission driving around our old neighborhood and visiting some friends. It was a good day, full of laughter and hope. That night I took her to the hospital and chatted with those who would be entrusted with my bride during the weeks to come. When it was time for me to go, she walked me down to the lobby. It was so hard to say good-bye. I wanted to be with her but could not. When I left, I drove past her twice to catch a glimpse of her lonely, frightened face as she braved an uncertain future. We both cried as we watched the distance and love between us grow.

Cindy was going to have to spend many days in isolation after the treatment began because her immune system would be severely weakened and she would be vulnerable to most of those common germs that exist all around us. For healthy people, these germs might cause only an uncomfortable cold. For Cindy, they would be certain death. We decided that it would be best if I returned home and took care of household business and the children while she continued with the ABMT. Cindy's family would be there every day to see her through the ordeal. I returned every two weeks to check on her progress and called her every day.

The ABMT is very hard on the recipient. Cindy was very nearly taken to the threshold of death. She lost her hair again, and her sight temporarily failed as the high-dose chemotherapy worked its good and bad on her. Her face and body puffed up, and she was so terribly sick. All I could do was provide love, sympathy, and comfort. But it was so hard to see her suffer so much. Watching a loved one suffer is the worst thing you can go through.

By Thanksgiving, she had recovered enough to be able to leave the hospital for a day. On this trip, I brought the kids. It was the most wonderful Thanksgiving we ever had.

More good news followed on the next day when we found out that Cindy could remain at Linda and Greg's. She was required to make regular visits to the hospital, but she was still able to stay at a home with loved ones. I continued to make visits as often as I could. Cindy, like the trouper that she was, made remarkable progress and grew stronger and stronger. She was my fighter. Never had she complained or voiced fear. A joke was her sword and her shield. Sometimes, however, during those quiet moments together, she would hold me and ask if I thought everything would be all right. I would truthfully answer yes. I did believe that the worst was behind us.

Just before Christmas, she was given permission to come home. We had had a lot of good Christmases together, but nothing could compare to having Cindy home and on the road to complete recovery. It was a family Christmas with our whole family together again.

. . . .
More insurance battles

When we settled with the insurance company, we had agreed to dismiss the lawsuit and pay our own attorneys' fees. However, even before

Cindy came home, the company wanted our attorneys to get us to sign a release document that would prevent us from filing any future lawsuits against them. It resembled a general release, without specific dates or parameters. This was the first time that Cindy and I were told of this though even our attorney claimed we had agreed to sign a release. The preauthorization sent to Cindy's hospital said nothing about a settlement, nor was there anything else in writing.

By the time Cindy was able to come home, attorneys' fees were taking most of the money collected by the fund-raiser. We could not afford to keep paying lawyers for a document that essentially benefited only the insurance company. We had been lied to, ignored, and generally treated so badly by the company that we just didn't trust the situation, no matter how innocent it looked. We let our attorneys go and considered the matter closed.

After that, we received a letter from the insurance company's attorneys telling us that Cindy and I were expected to hire another attorney to arrange the signing of the settlement agreement. I wrote back that we were not hiring more attorneys and that we were representing ourselves. I tried to negotiate with them and requested that they put the exact terms of the settlement payment into their agreement, i.e., that they would pay for all of Cindy's hospital stay. They refused.

The company attorneys continued to call and write us, expecting us to sign the agreement. At one point, they even tried withholding the medical payments they had promised until we signed a settlement. The irony of this was that just before they cut off our medical payments, Cindy and I had almost decided to sign the agreement just to alleviate the stress the situation was causing. But we weren't going to be blackmailed into signing anything. Cindy and I didn't trust anyone just then, the insurance company least of all.

The worst part of this was the stress they put us under, especially Cindy. I think this period was nearly as bad as the threat of cancer was. We had many sleepless nights worrying about what we should do. We finally closed the case ourselves by filing a dismissal notice stating that a settlement agreement was not part of the dismissal. We even enclosed the letter in which they said they would stop payment until we signed. At this point, the company backed off. To this day, I don't understand why this settlement was so important, since they were already protected by special-interest laws.

The battle with the insurance company took its toll on Cindy. It's extremely difficult to recover from a major illness when you're being hounded and harassed about something you cannot fully understand. Still, she somehow managed to rally and grew stronger once again. She helped start a local support group to help other cancer victims. Her hair grew back, along with her spirits. We even signed up for a cruise to Alaska, something Cindy had always wanted. Life was good once again.

Our good fortune was short-lived. The cough came back. Once again, my dear wife and friend was told that she was going to die. The doctor in Iowa told us that the ABMT had come too late. He explained that conventional chemotherapy kills the easy cancer cells and leaves the hardy ones behind, and these in turn divide and evolve into cancer cells that are resistant to treatment. She simply had been forced to be on conventional chemotherapy too long, and her cancer had become resistant, if not immune, to treatment. There was no more hope, no more miracles. All that could be done now was to begin conventional chemotherapy treatments again and hope that they could prolong her life.

Would Cindy have been cured had the ABMT treatment come sooner? Did the stress of suing the insurance company and dealing with the settlement agreement also harm her chances of recovery? There is no firm answer to these questions. But the insurance company and the Office of Personnel Management did steal, without any doubt, at least two or three years of life from my bride, and, quite possibly, the rest of an even longer life.

. . . .

No more miracles

Now we had finally come to that point when I, our children, her relatives, and her friends would be forced to watch Cindy slowly die. It was made harder because most of the time she did not look or act sick; she was always so bright, so positive, filled to overflowing with energy. She insisted on working and going on with her life as if nothing were wrong. She even laughed when her doctor suggested she get bottled oxygen in our home. If cancer was going to take her, it would not do so without a fight.

The disease that would take her from us was relentless, and, despite her iron will, it managed to take its toll on her. At times, it seemed to consume her minute by minute. Finally, she had to admit that she really needed oxygen. With the oxygen supply, she was able to build herself up again and still work and resume fairly normal activities.

Her first major setback came when she admitted to me that she could no longer work full days and wanted to know if she could work half days for a while. This was so typical of Cindy—to be more concerned for others than she was for herself. She worked half days for two weeks before she admitted that she could no longer go on. She wanted to stay home "for a while, until my strength comes back."

The point when I finally knew that I was really going to lose her came when we returned home from one of her Friday chemo treatments and she was too weak to walk on her own into our house. I had to carry her into the house and upstairs to our bedroom. She was so ashamed that she could not do it herself. In her indomitable fashion, she chastised herself by calling herself lazy.

Her decline was frighteningly fast after that. There was always that persistent cough, day and night; she could not escape the monster nipping at her heels. We turned our bedroom into the central gathering place of the house. We put in a TV, and family meals were taken there. Cindy weakened in body but not in spirit. She still laughed easily and joked about everything, even her oncoming death. She worried about money and what we would do without her but never about what would happen to her when she died.

The one thing she made clear was that she did not want to die at home. She was adamant about this point. When the time came, she wanted it to happen in a hospital.

On her last Friday on earth, I helped her to the car and drove her to her once-a-week chemo treatment. It was very difficult for her to travel at this point. Even with oxygen, she labored to breathe, and without it, she suffered much more. It was immediately clear to the doctor that the chemo was doing no good. There was nothing more that could be done medically. Cindy pressed him to say how much time she had left. He told her that it was difficult, if not impossible, to know with any certainty. She insisted, and he reluctantly guessed at perhaps another two weeks. The last hope that Cindy had clung to was that she would live long enough to make her cruise to Alaska. Now she knew she would not make it in this life, and it broke her heart.

We both knew that this was it. I had this feeling that she would never come home again, so I tried to get her to go home with me, desperately hoping that this would prolong her life. But she knew that this was her time, and she insisted that she be placed in the hospital "for a few days just to get some rest."

She went into the hospital on July 5, 1991. I spent as much time as I could with her. On Sunday, I brought the children in, and we spent our last day as a family together. She was dying and she knew it, but she still joked with the nurses, me, and the kids. She could barely breathe, but still she laughed and would always smile. I took our kids home that evening and came back alone to spend the evening with her.

. . . .
Cindy says goodbye

That last evening, she just looked at me and smiled and said, "Talk to me." I asked what about, and she would only repeat, "Talk to me." She could barely breathe at this point. So I talked. I talked about our good times together, the fun, our accomplishments, our joy, our love. I recalled humorous events and repeated the jokes I could remember. I talked about our friends, family, children, anything I could think of. Cindy listened quietly, smiling, always looking into my face, her blue eyes brimming with the life that would soon leave her body.

The hospital announced that visiting hours were ending at 10:00 P.M. I had this feeling that I should spend the night with her. When I told her that I wanted to stay, she insisted strongly that I return home to the kids. I argued, but she was very firm about my leaving. Looking back now, I think we both knew what was going to happen. Cindy knew it was her time to go, and she wanted to spare me the burden of seeing her die. I reluctantly kissed her good-bye, and we held hands as I told her how much I loved her. She was able to sit up and smile at me as I left her room.

Part of me was grateful to return home. I was physically and emotionally drained and needed to get some sleep. I guess I knew that I'd never see Cindy alive again, but I could not admit it and counted on another two weeks. I planned to return in the morning to spend the day with her again. It was after 11:00 P.M. by the time I got home, so I went right to bed, falling asleep the instant my head hit the pillow.

The phone rang at 3:00 A.M., and Cindy's nurse informed me that Cindy was having a bad time and asked if I could come. I quickly dressed and started the forty-minute drive to the hospital. I was driving past the airport at 3:20 A.M. when it felt like an ocean wave passed over the car. It did not affect the car, but I felt it very clearly as a real, tangible force. I started to cry, but, at the time, could not admit what I had just experienced. The few people I've told about this usually give me a sympathetic but skeptical look that tells me they think they understand what I'm going through and that I'm merely a grieving widower grasping at emotional shadows. But I can tell you this without hesitation, even many months after Cindy's death—it was real, as real as anything on earth. And it did not happen just to me. Some of Cindy's friends experienced something similar at precisely the same instant. Cindy had to leave us, but she did not go until she said good-bye.

When I got to the hospital, my Cindy was gone.

It took a long time to say good-bye that morning. Perhaps it will take the rest of my life to finish saying it. But there is another side to this place we think we know. There will be a time in that other place when Cindy and I will meet again. If I ever had any doubts about life after death, they're gone now.

The sun was up by the time I returned to my car. The world was busy getting ready for the new day, blissfully unaware of the tragic event that had just happened while most of them were still in bed. I went home to tell the kids what had happened and make arrangements for the funeral.

We survived the aftermath somehow, in a numb, dazed sort of way. Eventual recovery will take a long, long time, if ever.

Since Cindy died, I've had many dreams about her, some pleasant, some nightmare replays of our ordeal. On three occasions, however, she came back to me. The first two times she merely walked into my sleep and smiled and watched me, much the same way she did at the hospital on her last day. On the third visit, she spoke to me. I know the difference between my dreams and her visits. Her visits were real. I don't push the issue. I write this now only because some of you reading this will be helped by knowing this. I merely offer what I know to be true.

I've come to believe that our existence here is some kind of education. We were sent here to learn as much as we can, to learn compassion, wisdom, charity to others, love, and all of those other things that seem to be learned best the hard way, through hands-on experience and time. Perhaps God was able to give us everything except wisdom.

I don't profess to understand the nature of God any more than I did before. My religious training and education have failed me. My faith in a higher order, though, is much stronger. Even the pain and suffering we see and experience must serve some purpose we cannot possibly understand— yet. I believe more and more that we here in this place are not meant to understand too much. We must use our time to learn instead. Perhaps we're here to find and experience love.

There is a crossing over when we die, and we take what we have learned, what we have gained, with us to that place. We will meet again those who have left before us. I doubt during our lifetimes that we'll ever really know any more than this. We probably don't need to know any more than this.

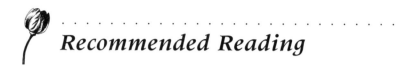

Recommended Reading

The following list is not meant to be exhaustive; it contains those books that the contributors found helpful in dealing with various aspects of their breast cancer.

Autobiographies

First You Cry, Betty Rollin, 1976

It's Always Something, Gilda Radner, 1989

Last Wish, Betty Rollin, 1985

Life Wish, Jill Ireland, 1987

The Race Is Run One Step at a Time, Nancy G. Brinker, 1995

Cancer

Beauty and Cancer, Diane D. Noyes, 1988

Breast Cancer: What Every Woman Should Know, Paul Rodriguez, M.D.

Breast Self-Examination, Albert Milan, M.D.

Cancer . . . There's Hope (1981) and *Fighting Cancer* (1985), Annette
       and Richard Bloch, both available from: Cancer Connection,
       4410 Main Street, Kansas City, Missouri, 64111

Cancer as a Turning Point, Lawerence LeShan

The Cancer Survivors and How They Did It, Judith Glassman, 1983

Dr. Susan Love's Breast Book, Susan M. Love, M.D., 1990

Every Woman's Guide to Breast Cancer, Vicki L. Seltzer, M.D.

Keeping Abreast, Kerry A. McGinn, R.N.

Love, Medicine, and Miracles, Bernie S. Siegel, M.D., 1986

Man to Man: When the Woman You Love Has Breast Cancer,
    Andy Murcia and Bob Stewart

No Less a Woman, Deborah H. Kahane, M.S.W., 1990

Peace, Love, and Healing, Bernie S. Siegel, M.D., 1989

The Race Is Run One Step at a Time, Nancy G. Brinker, 1995

Women Talk about Breast Cancer, Amy Gross and Dee Ito, 1990

You Can Fight for Your Life: Emotional Factors in the Causation of Cancer,
    Lawerence LeShan, 1977

Your Breasts: A Complete Guide, Jerome F. Levy, M.D.

Family/Relationships

The Continuum Concept: Allowing Human Nature to Work Successfully,
    Jean Lieflof

The Family, John Bradshaw, 1988

Father Loss, Elyce Wakerman, 1984

Making Peace with Your Parents, Harold H. Bloomfield

My Mother, Myself, Nancy Friday

What You Can Feel, You Can Heal, John Gray, 1984

Grief/Death

Coming Back: Rebuilding Lives after Crisis and Loss,
    Ann Kaiser Stearns, 1988

The Courage to Grieve, Judy Tatelbaum, 1980

A Gift of Hope: How We Survive Our Tragedies, Robert Veninga, 1985

A Grief Observed, C.S. Lewis, 1961

Grieving: How to Go On Living When Someone You Love Dies,
    Therese Rando, 1988

How to Survive the Loss of a Love, Melba Colgrove,
    Harold Bloomfield, & Peter McWilliam, 1977

I Never Know What to Say, Nina Horrmann Donnelly, 1987

To Live Until We Say Goodbye, Elizabeth Kubler-Ross, 1978

Who Dies? An Investigation of Conscious Living and Conscious Dying,
Stephen Levine, 1982

Self-Help/Special Issues

Anatomy of an Illness, Norman Cousins, 1981

Anger: The Misunderstood Emotion, Carol Tavris

Are You There, God? It's Me, Margaret, Judy Blume, 1970

Celebrate the Temporary, Clyde Reid, 1974

Celebrate Yourself, Dorothy Corkville Briggs

Codependent No More, Melodie Beattie

Creative Visualization, Shakti Gawain, 1982

Dance of Anger, Harriet Lerner, Ph.D.

Every Woman's Emotional Well-Being, Carol Tavris

Fat Is a Feminist Issue, I and II, Susie Orbach

Feeling Good: The New Mood Therapy, David Burns, 1981

Getting Well Again, O. Carl and Stephanie Simonton, 1980

Healing the Child Within, Charles Whitfield, 1987

Human Options, Norman Cousins

I Ain't Much, Baby—But I'm All I've Got, Jess Lair, Ph.D., 1978

Jane Brody's Good Food Book, Jane Brody

Jane Brody's Nutrition Book, Jane Brody

Life Is Uncertain . . . Eat Dessert First!, S. Gordon and H. Brecher,1990

Life 101, John-Roger and Peter McWilliams, 1990

Living, Loving, and Learning, Leo Buscaglia, Ph.D.

Living Beyond Fear: Coping with the Emotional Aspects of Life-Threatening Illness, Jeanne Segal, Ph.D., 1989

Living Through Personal Crisis, Ann Kaiser Stearns, 1984

Love, Leo Buscaglia, Ph.D.

Man's Search for Meaning, Viktor Frankl, 1963

Meditations for Women Who Do Too Much, Anne Wilson Schaef, 1990

Minding the Body, Mending the Mind, Joan Borysenko, 1987

My Body, My Decision, Lindsey Curtis, M.D.

Necessary Losses, Judith Viorst, 1986

New Our Bodies, Ourselves, Boston Women's Health Book Collective

Once a Month, Katherine Dalton

Opening Up: The Healing Power of Confiding in Others,
      James W. Pennebaker, 1990

Our Ground Time Here Will Be Brief, Maxine Kumin, 1982

Passages, Gail Sheehy, 1976

Pathfinders, Gail Sheehy, 1981

The Power Within You, John-Roger McWilliams

The Road Less Traveled, M. Scott Peck, M.D., 1978

The Superwoman Syndrome, Marjorie H. Shaevitz, 1984

When Bad Things Happen to Good People, Harold Kushner, 1981

Women and Fatigue, Holly Atkinson, M.D.

You Can Heal Your Life, Louise L. Hay, 1984

You Can't Afford the Luxury of a Negative Thought,
      John-Roger and Peter McWilliams, 1990

Special Interest

Cancer Ward, Alexander Solzhenitsyn

Drama of the Gifted Child, Alice Miller, Ph.D.

Full Catastrophe Living, Jon Kabot-Zinn, 1990

The Macrobiotic Approach to Cancer, Michio Kushi & E/W Foundation

Mind as Healer, Mind as Slayer, Kenneth Pellitier, 1977

The Prophet, Kahlil Gibran, 1923

Raising Children with Success, Steven Glen

Raising Responsible Children, Steven Glen

Recalled by Life, Anthony J. Sattilaro, M.D., 1982

Spence & Lila, Bobbie Ann Mason

Understanding, Jane Nelson

Zen Macrobiotic Cooking, Michel Abehsera